DOWN AND DIRTY

DOWN AND DIRTY

THE ESSENTIAL TRAINING GUIDE FOR OBSTACLE RACES AND MUD RUNS

MATT B. DAVIS

FOREWORD BY SCOTT KENEALLY,
DIRECTOR OF *RISE OF THE SUFFERFESTS*

Fair Winds Press
100 Cummings Center, Suite 406L
Beverly, MA 01915

fairwindspress.com • bodymindbeautyhealth.com

First published in the USA in 2014 by
Fair Winds Press, a member of
Quarto Publishing Group USA Inc.
100 Cummings Center
Suite 406-L
Beverly, MA 01915-6101
www.fairwindspress.com
Visit www.bodymindbeautyhealth.com. It's your personal guide to a happy, healthy, and
extraordinary life!

18 17 16 15 14   1 2 3 4 5

ISBN: 978-1-59233-599-2

Digital edition published in 2014
eISBN: 978-1-62788-022-0

Library of Congress Cataloging-in-Publication Data available

Cover and book design by Megan Jones Design
Cover image: Brent Doscher/Nuvision Action Image

Printed and bound in China

Know your limits. The authors and Quarto Publishing Group USA Inc. assume no liability
for accidents happening to, or injuries sustained by, readers who engage in the activities
described in this book.

TO MY MOM AND DAD, ANNA, JENNI, AND RACHAEL

CONTENTS

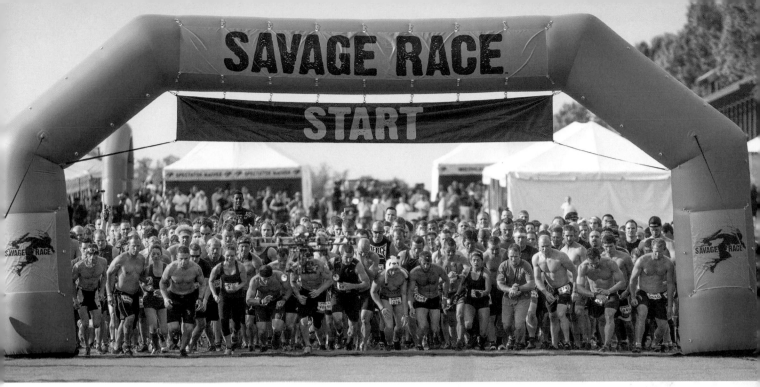

▲ *Here we go.*

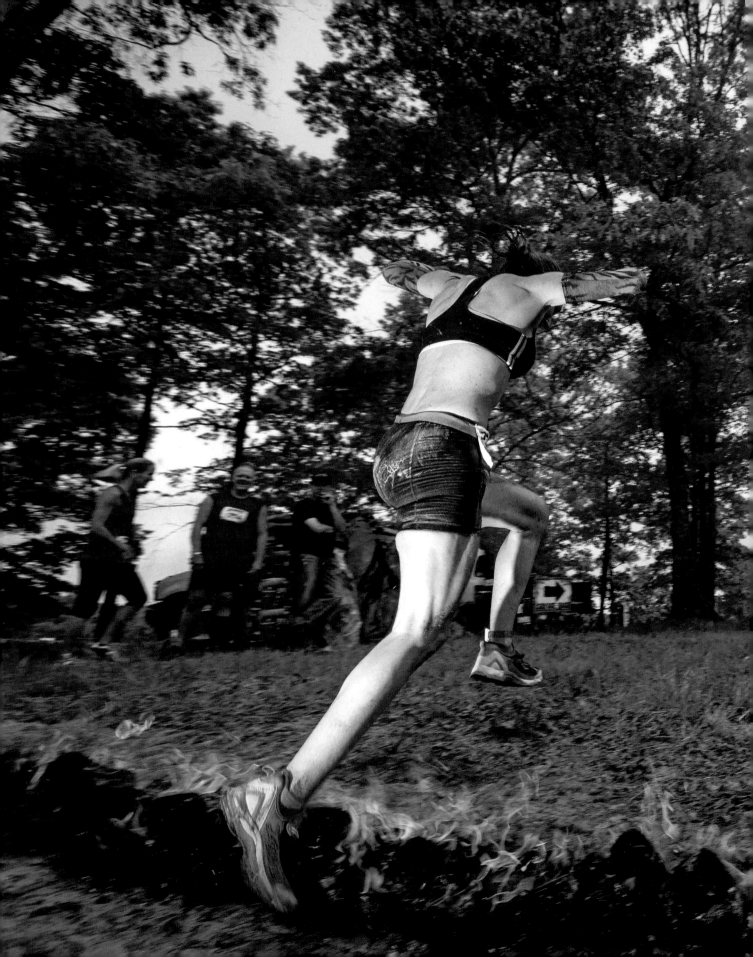

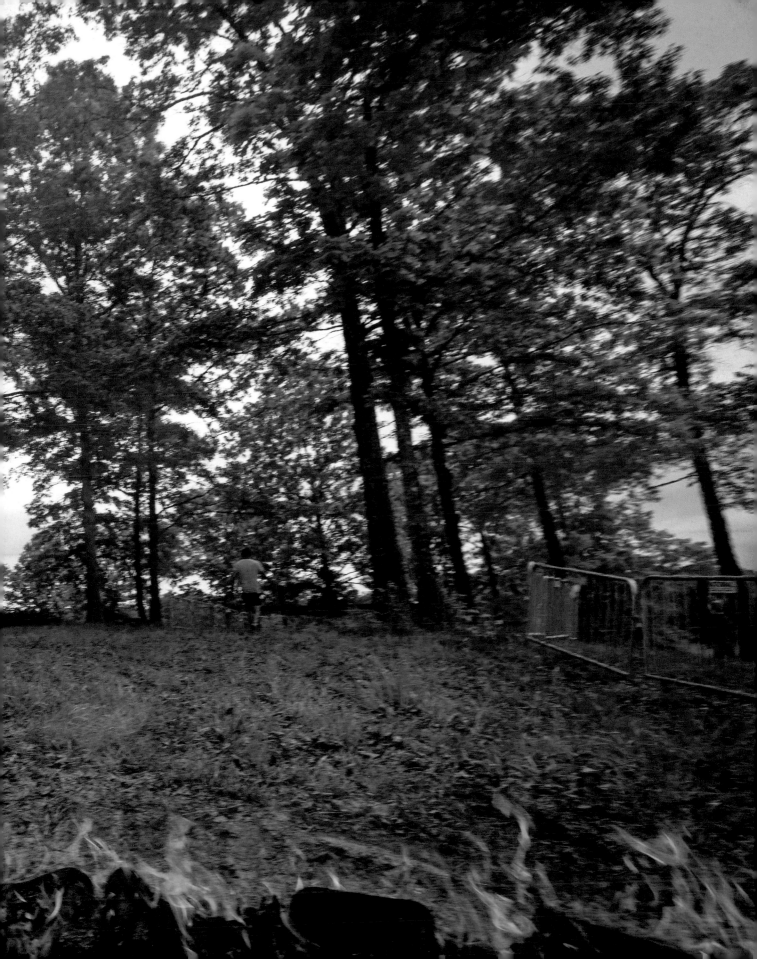

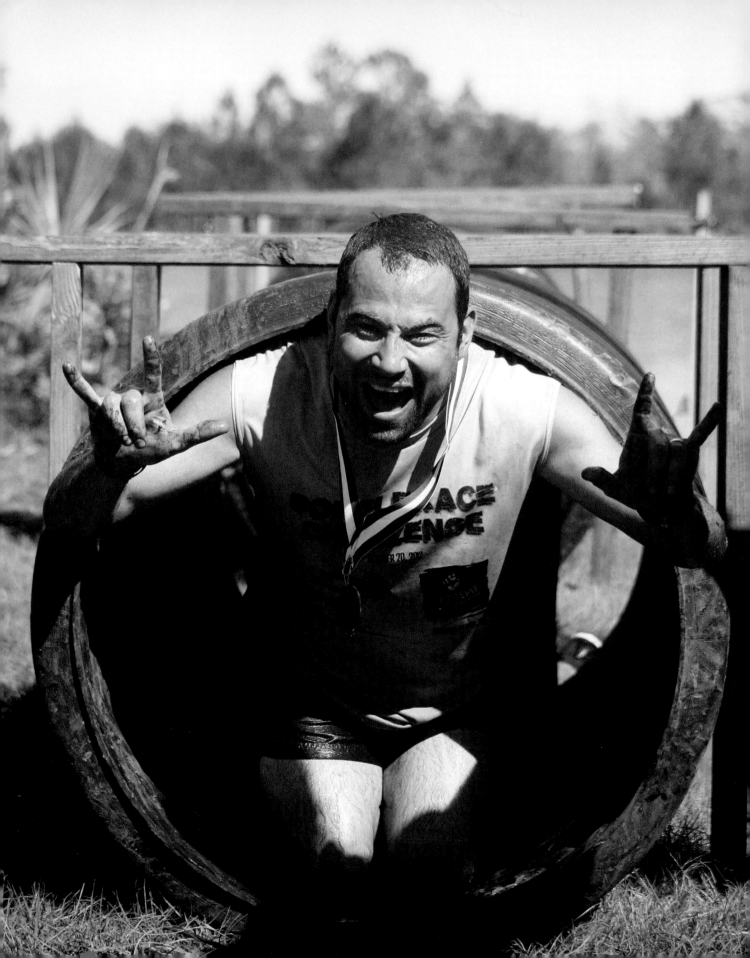

FOREWORD

Shortly after *Outside* magazine published my first feature on obstacle racing, a cover story about the scandalous origins of Tough Mudder, Matt B. Davis reached out. Like an OCR fan boy, he enthusiastically picked my brain for any details or dirt left on the editing room floor, and then asked to interview me on his podcast. At the time, I was holding out for an interview with a more—how to put this?—*professional* outfit. Say, *60 Minutes*, for instance. So I politely declined, though this did little to deter him from asking. Again and again, again and again. The man is nothing if not persistent—think Cujo—and this rabid fanaticism has helped Matt become the most connected journalist in the OCR world. Thanks to a weekly podcast with a broad spectrum of athletes and industry insiders, and in-depth reporting for Obstacle Racing Media, Matt has gained the trust and respect of the community. So it made sense that he would land a contract to write this book. But his real stroke of genius wasn't the book deal itself, it was Matt's ability to "write a book" without really writing at all. Thanks to a mix of arm twists and guilt trips, he managed to outsource half of the work to others. Smart, right? Brilliant, actually.

No wonder they call him the Wizard of Obs.

Scott Keneally—Author of Playing Dirty *and director of* Rise of the Sufferfests

◄ *The author, commonly known as Cujo to interviewees.*

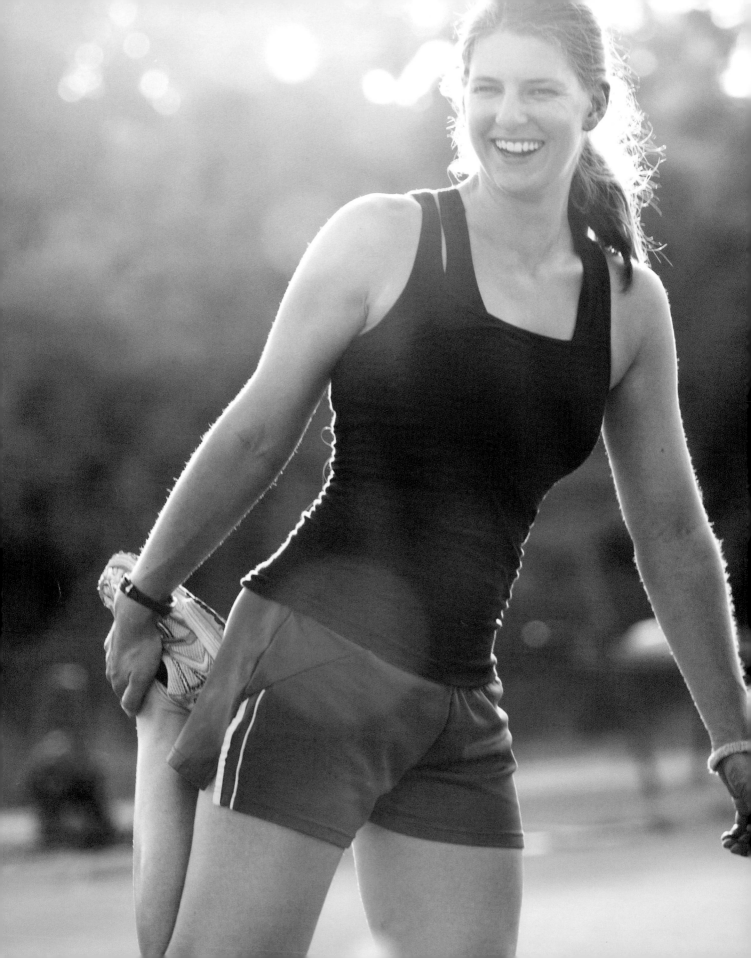

PREFACE

Y ou've seen pictures of friends muddy, bruised, and bloody, wading through ice-cold, blue-tinged water, chest deep in mud, or painfully trudging through a curtain of electrical wires. Despite their clear suffering, the photos taken at the finish line show your friends smiling broadly. Your coworkers come in to work on a Monday with large medals around their necks or orange headbands on their foreheads, beaming with pride. They can't wait to tell you about the pain they endured, the barriers they overcame, and the laughs they had.

Obstacle course racing and mud runs have exploded in popularity in recent years. Though they began just a few years ago with a handful of military boot camp–style events taken on by the brave, stupid—or both, obstacle racing is now a worldwide phenomenon. Experts are predicting it will soon be a $1 billion industry, and the participant numbers could top the 4 million mark.

The obstacle course racing world is everywhere you look, and it goes far beyond the mud pit. The news media constantly features stories on obstacle course racing, including national outlets from the *Wall Street Journal* to *60 Minutes*. Outdoor gear, clothing, and shoe companies sponsor races and market their products and advertisements to obstacle course racers.

This book offers in-depth, expert advice on how to train and prepare for mud runs, obstacle course races, and endurance events. Having participated in more than forty races, I've acquired a ton of knowledge in the past few years, and I can't wait to share it with beginners and

◀ *Get ready for a whole new kind of race.*

advanced obstacle course racers alike. I've also tapped the vast knowledge of experts in the industry, including elite athletes and specialists such as Death Race winner Olof Dallner, World's Toughest Mudder Amelia Boone, Spartan Pro Team Racer Alec Blenis, and obstacle builder extraordinaire Rob Butler.

Two types of people will benefit from this book. The first are folks who have never done an obstacle course race and are looking to find out where to begin. This book is going to help you get there in a relatively short time.

You may be someone who goes to the gym once a week (or less). You probably have not run more than 1 mile (1.6 km) in the past ten to fifteen years. You may not be able to do more than two pull-ups in a row. No problem. You're exactly where I was a few short years ago when I signed up for my first Tough Mudder. I hadn't run more than a mile or lifted a weight since middle school. This book will get you at least five times more prepared than I was before I tackled that first 10- to 12-mile (16.1- to 19.3-km) obstacle course race.

The second group that will benefit from this book is the more experienced racers who are looking to gain an edge by reading and incorporating ideas about training, form, and diet from some top elite athletes and experts in the sport. My experience in the past few years includes running more than forty obstacle races and producing more than seventy podcast episodes about obstacle racing. In those episodes, I interviewed more than fifty athletes and more than twenty race directors. I asked many of those racers and directors to contribute their expertise for this book. They offer their advice on running, training, CrossFit WODs (Workout of the Day), nutrition, hydration, gear, and more.

"Get faster, go farther, and prepare to conquer any obstacle."

This book will cover a variety of topics and get you more prepared and involved than any other book of its kind. You'll get some history and learn about some of the founding fathers of the sport—before it was even a sport. If you're a beginner, this book will get you off the couch to run your first mile. It will get you prepared to climb those first ropes and crawl under the first set of barbed wire. For the more experienced racer, this book includes some advanced techniques and other more serious (and dangerous) ventures. (Death Race, anyone?) For the newbie and advanced alike, the industry's top athletes will teach you how to get faster,

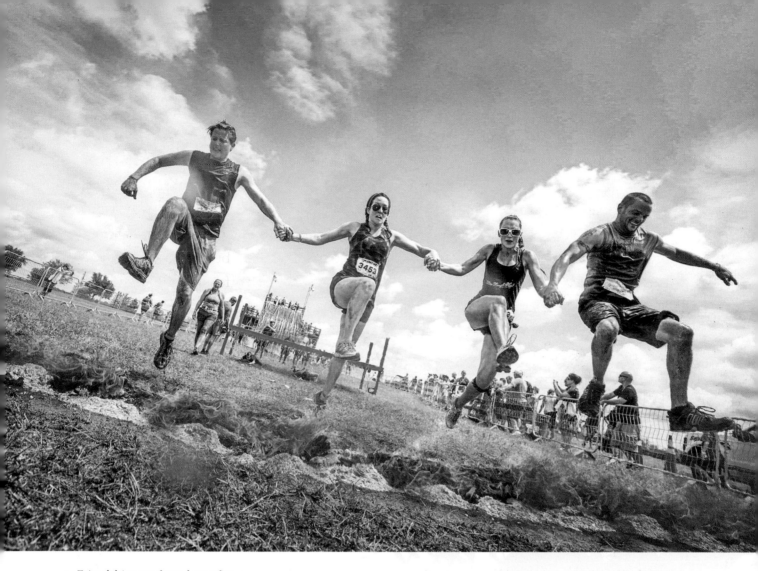

▲ *Friendships are forged over fire.*

go farther, and prepare to conquer any obstacle. You'll also find resources to help you find more folks like you who are currently training for these races and looking to form a team.

Here's your opportunity to learn from the best in the business how to improve your ability to go over walls, under wires, and through mud and fire. My hope is that you find what I have found by choosing to participate in this new and growing sport: a way to push your body and mind to places you never thought you could go, the freedom and laughter that you experienced as a ten year old by losing yourself in an obstacle course, and the amazing friendships you'll create with other racers.

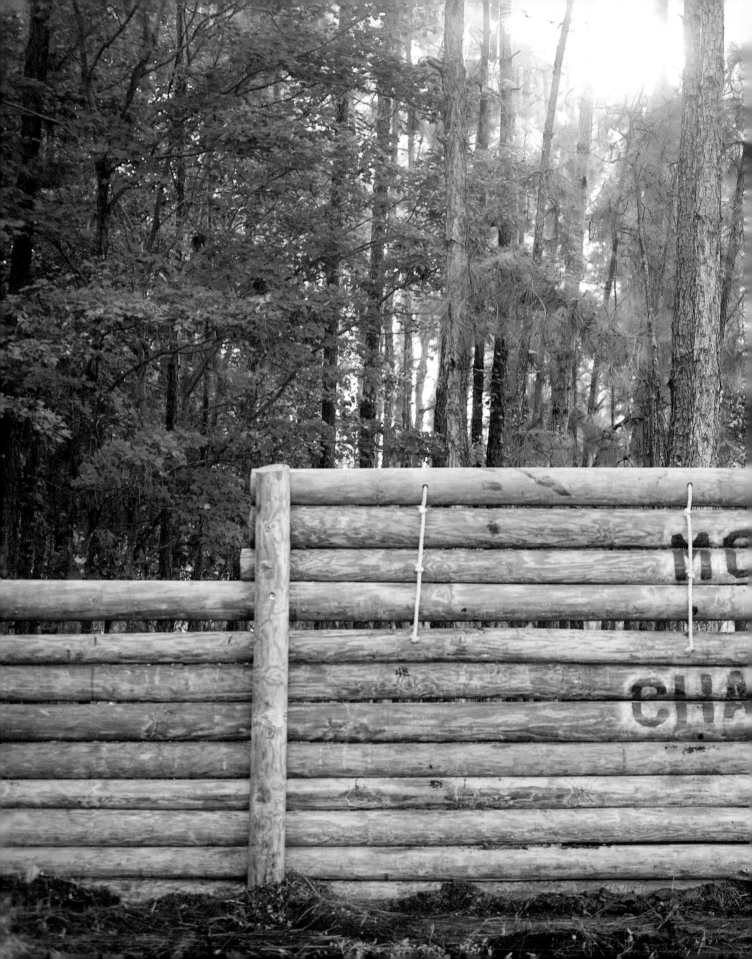

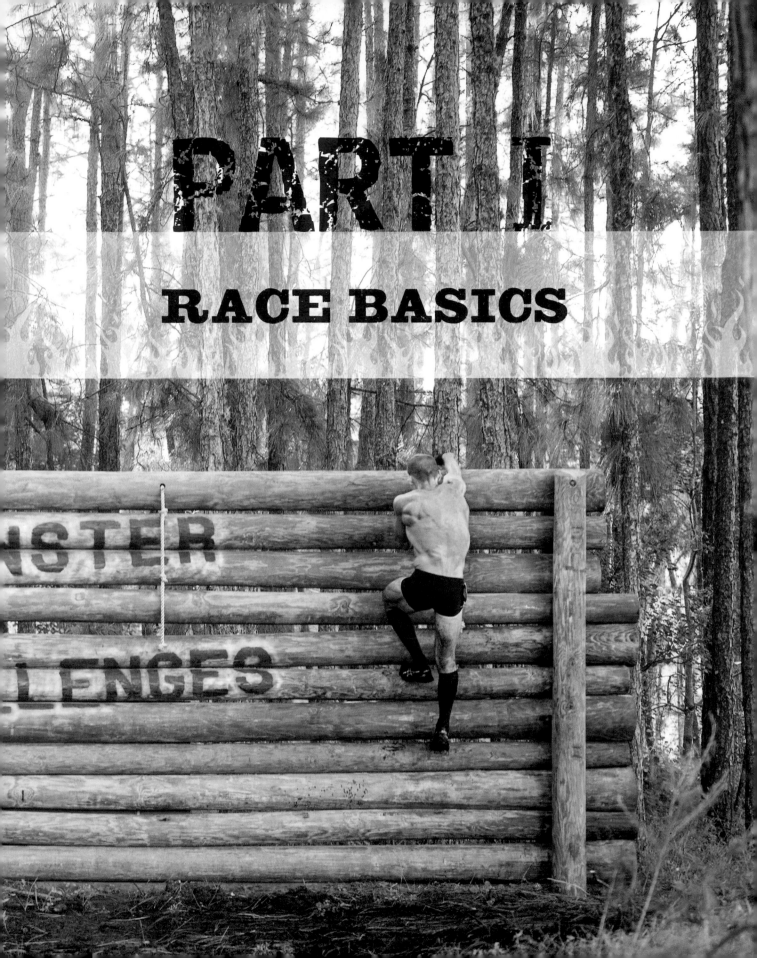

PART II

RACE BASICS

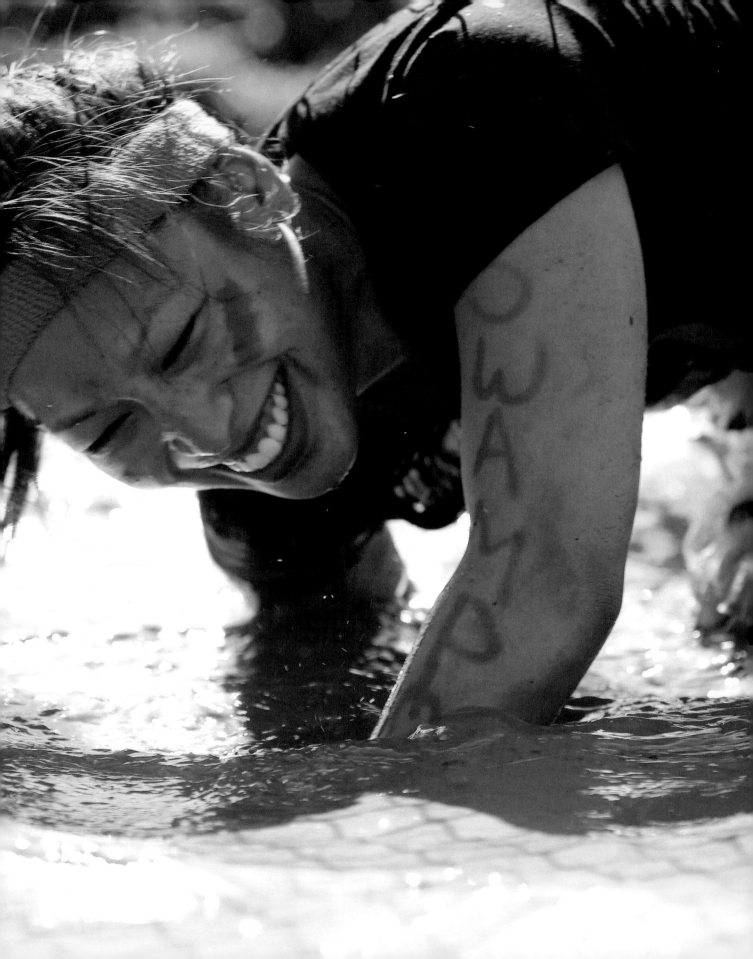

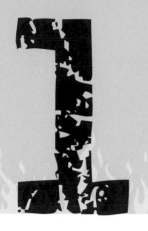

THE HISTORY OF OBSTACLE COURSE RACING

If you've purchased this book, or if you're currently reading it in the bookstore because you have time to kill, you're most likely well aware of what obstacle course racing (OCR) is. However, what good would I be in presenting this book to you without laying out a basic definition of OCR?

Per Wikipedia, "Obstacle racing is a sport in which a competitor, traveling on foot, must overcome various physical challenges (obstacles). They combine mud and trail runs designed to result in mental and physical collapse. Obstacles include, but are not limited to, climbing over walls, carrying heavy objects, traversing bodies of water, crawling under barbed wire, and jumping through fire. Many obstacles are similar to those used in military training, whilst others are unique to obstacle racing and are employed throughout the course to test endurance, strength, speed, and dexterity."

Obstacle course racing can be traced back to the ancient Greeks, who used a form of obstacle courses to train for combat. Today, branches of many militaries use confidence courses as a way to train their soldiers. Steeplechase, (which was born in 1860 and later became an event in the modern Olympics), had runners jumping over wooden hurdles and through water obstacles. Basically, as long as people could run, they've wanted to jump over, on top of, and through things along the way to test individual athleticism, to compete against each other, and to simply have fun.

You can spend hours scouring the Internet or the library (remember those?) to find specific facts on what the early

◄ *Muddy moments like this have been happening for longer than you may think.*

races looked like. Perhaps you could even find out the first person who said, "Hey, instead of just a foot race, let's see who can go through that thing and over that stuff, the fastest and the best."

For the purposes of this book, we'll jump ahead to a recent century to see how modern OCR was born.

In 1987, Billy Wilson, a.k.a. Mr. Mouse, created an event called Tough Guy in the U.K., which featured huge walls to climb and mud to crawl through, and was the first event to force people into frigid water and subject participants to electric shocks.

Mr. Mouse was very proud to tell me, "I created Tough Guy as the Fun Run that combined fun and fear. No timing chips were needed, no set measured distance, and no prizes. Runners encountered Terror Miles, Brutal Wooded Hillsides, Farm Much, Cattle Electric Fences, Tree Climbing, and Swinging Ropes. We also created the system of numbering racers with a marker pen because paper numbers got destroyed."

In 1993, Camp Pendleton, in California, put on a basic confidence course with some extra mud thrown in and invited people to run it. Sixty-five people, mostly military personnel and their families,

turned up, and the event was considered a success. It's now known as the World Famous Mud Run.

Bob Babbitt, an experienced runner and triathlete, was intrigued by the fun he had at an event called a "ride and tie." In the event, two runners are paired together, each team has a horse, and they leapfrog each other over the course of 28 miles (45.1 km), taking turns running or riding the horse. In 1999, Babbitt decided to replace the horse with a bike and add some obstacles and mud, and the Muddy Buddy was born in Oceanside, California.

All of these events were successful by their own measurements. They each continued, without any real national attention, year after year.

Then, in the latter half of the 2000s, three companies with slightly different philosophies came along and started a full-on OCR revolution. This movement is what led to the writing of this book.

Now let's talk about what has come to be known as the Big 3: the Tough Mudder, Warrior Dash, and Spartan Race.

▶ *Mud pits are some of the best posing opportunities.*

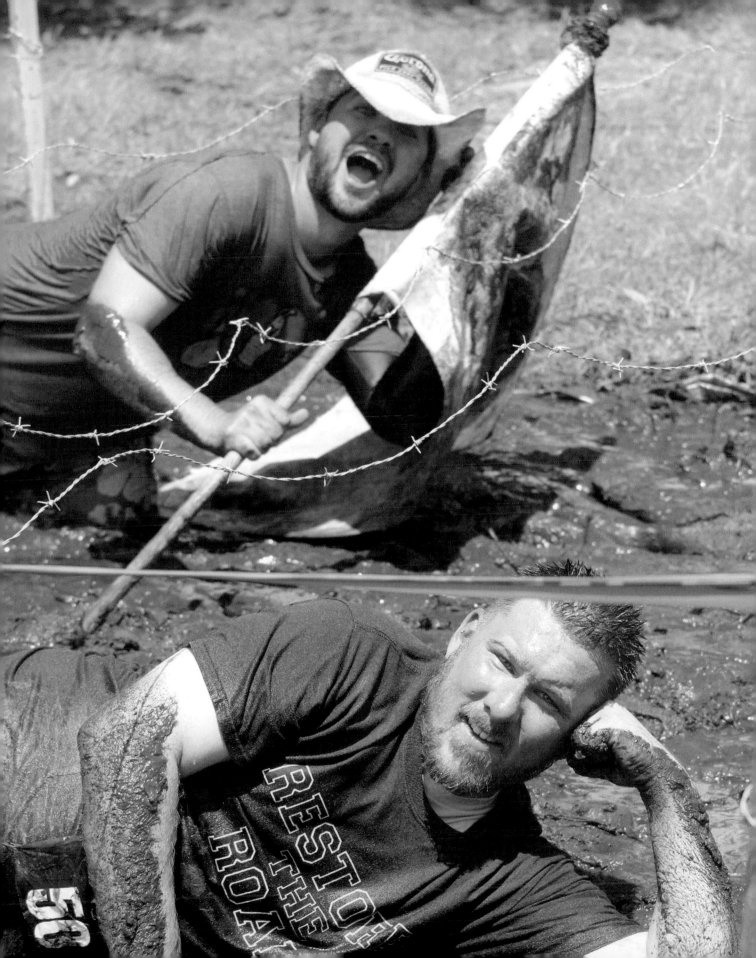

Tough Mudder

In 2010, Will Dean and Guy Livingstone were Harvard students from England who saw the success of the United Kingdom's Tough Guy and wanted to bring a form of it to the United States. With minimal investment, they put an event together in New Jersey. Will was quoted as saying, "I wanted to make something that was Ironman-meets-Burning Man, a test of all-around fitness, but in this fun, slightly quirky environment." Dean and Livingstone expected to get about 500 entrants. They got just less than 5,000. The videos from their first view events went viral, and people could not wait to sign up for future events. Execs at Tough Mudder have been quoted as saying, "Experience is the new luxury good; buying stuff doesn't make you happier."

Warrior Dash

In 2009, Warrior Dash came onto the scene with their first event in Illinois. Their idea was to ask weekend warriors to get off the couch and race through a 3-mile (4.8 km) course with some fun obstacles and lots of mud. When the racers crossed the finish line, they were given a Fred Flintstone–style warrior "helmet," a beer, and a king-size turkey leg. People couldn't wait to get *those* photos on Facebook. The next year, Warrior Dash held a dozen events nationwide.

Spartan Race

Joe DeSena and Andy Weinberg had been successful endurance athletes who had traveled the world doing all kinds of crazy adventures. The problem was that those events required lots of travel and time away from home. The events also required a large pocketbook, and only a certain demographic could compete. So in 2005, DeSena and Weinberg put on something known as the Death Race in their hometown of Pittsfield, Vermont. They wanted to test people's will, athleticism, and endurance in a way that no one had before, without having to travel halfway around the world. With no rules, course, or official start or end times, the Death Race attracted only the extremely brave/insane.

In 2010, DeSena and Weinberg set out to create an event with a similar intensity, but scaled down to a real 3- to 5-mile (4.8 to 8.1 km) obstacle race with an actual start and finish. DeSena and Weinberg can often be heard preaching the "gospel" of Spartan, which is basically the

▶ *The variety of physical challenges will require practice and patience, but the rewards will be sweet.*

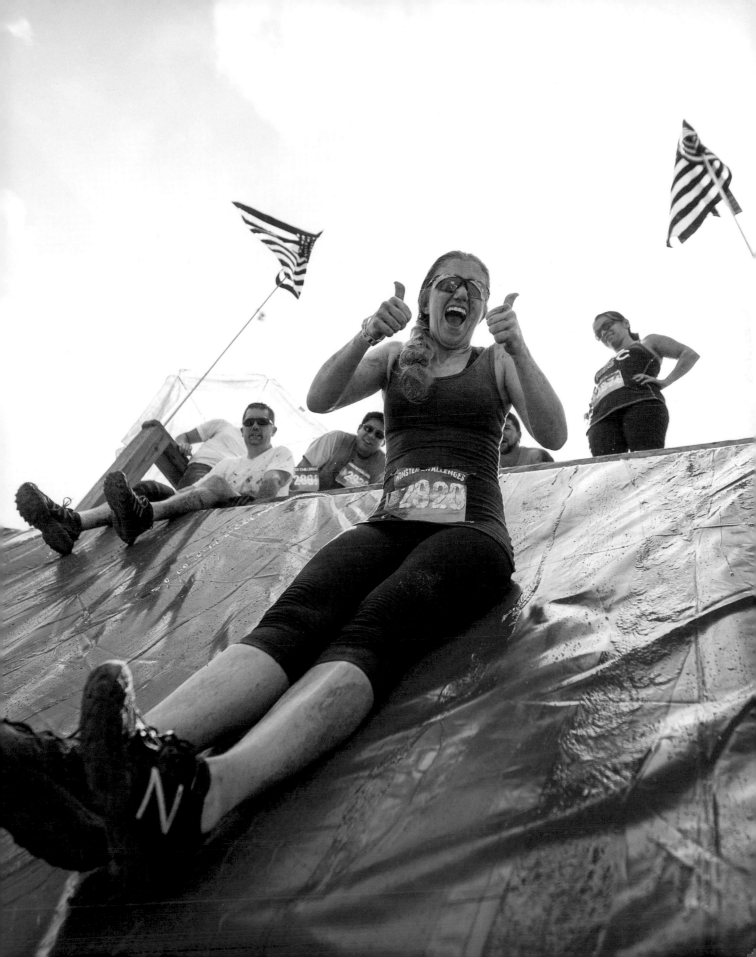

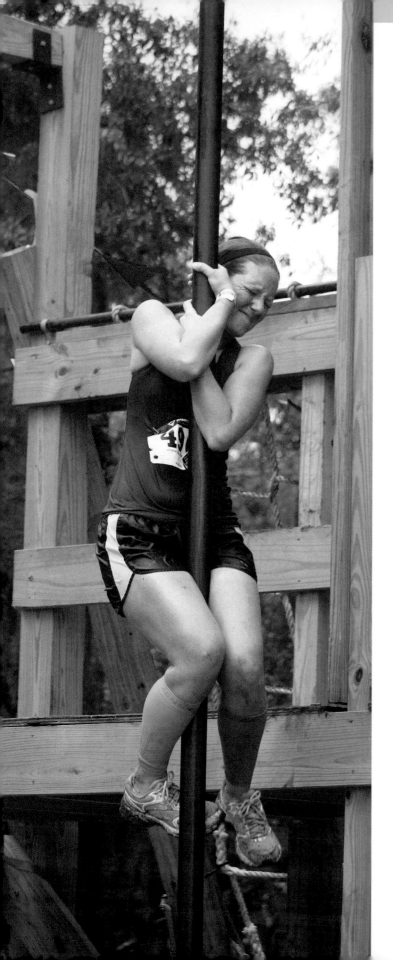

belief that in today's modern world, "everything is too easy," and we live in an "everyone-gets-a-medal" society. If you come to a Spartan philosophy, DeSena and Weinberg promise that "You will discover a sense of exhilaration and personal achievement that has eluded you in every other sport or endeavor, and you'll see yourself in an entirely new light."

Of the Big 3 events, the Spartan Race is the only one that times all racers and has penalties for not completing. Its organizers are proud of their promise that you'll be "ranked, timed, and judged."

These three races all became massive successes, and they each grew exponentially in their first two to three years. Every other day, it seemed, an article was written in a major publication about the world's fascination with getting dirty and pushing physical boundaries.

The organizers of these races set the bar with high production values, well-trained and enthusiastic staff and volunteers, obstacles that are extremely well-built, and lively festival areas with beer, food, and music. They quickly became the measuring stick for all the other events that sprang up in this wave of excitement.

◄ *Hold on tight.*

Obstacle Racing in the United Kingdom

The Tough Guy Challenge was the first official obstacle race worldwide, put together by Billy "Mr. Mouse" Wilson in Wolverhampton in 1987. (See page 20). It wasn't until 2009 that Spartan Race arrived. Spartan brought a new approach, with timed races and varied distances. What quickly followed was a flurry of races, like the Nuts Challenge and Total Warrior, each with a different presentation and challenges.

Tough Guy would later inspire two Harvard guys to start Tough Mudder in the U.S. For more on that intriguing and controversial tale, I highly recommend Scott Kenealy's article, "Playing Dirty" in *Outside* magazine (November 2012). Tough Mudder came to the U.K. with strong foundations, ready to really shake things up.

Today obstacle racing is booming. There are more than 80 different race organizations putting on events. Meanwhile, Mr. Mouse's course has grown and grown on its permanent site and now boasts more than 200 obstacles and up to 5,000 participants per event.

Obstacle Racing in Australia

In 2008, a bike and mountain race company called Maximum Adventure produced an event called the Tough Bloke Challenge. This race was inspired in part by U.K.'s Tough Guy and brought in about 500 participants. Maximum Adventure later added a less intense event they called simply "Mud Run."

A few years later, Warrior Dash made its way over from the United States, and a local company called The Stampede launched. A local favorite, The Stampede currently attracts 8,000 to 10,000 participants. In 2012, Tough Mudder exported its widely popular brand of racing and brought a staggering 20,000 participants to its early events.

In 2013, Spartan Race Australia launched. Spartan has not done as well as its American counterpart, attracting between 2,000 and 3,000 participants per race. Also in 2013, a league of elite obstacle athletes formed, but only includes about 150 racers.

The verdict is still out in Australia, as new races are popping up as quickly as other races are closing or failing to get off the ground. Meanwhile, Tough Mudder returns in 2014 with seven races, currently averaging 12,000 to 15,000 per event.

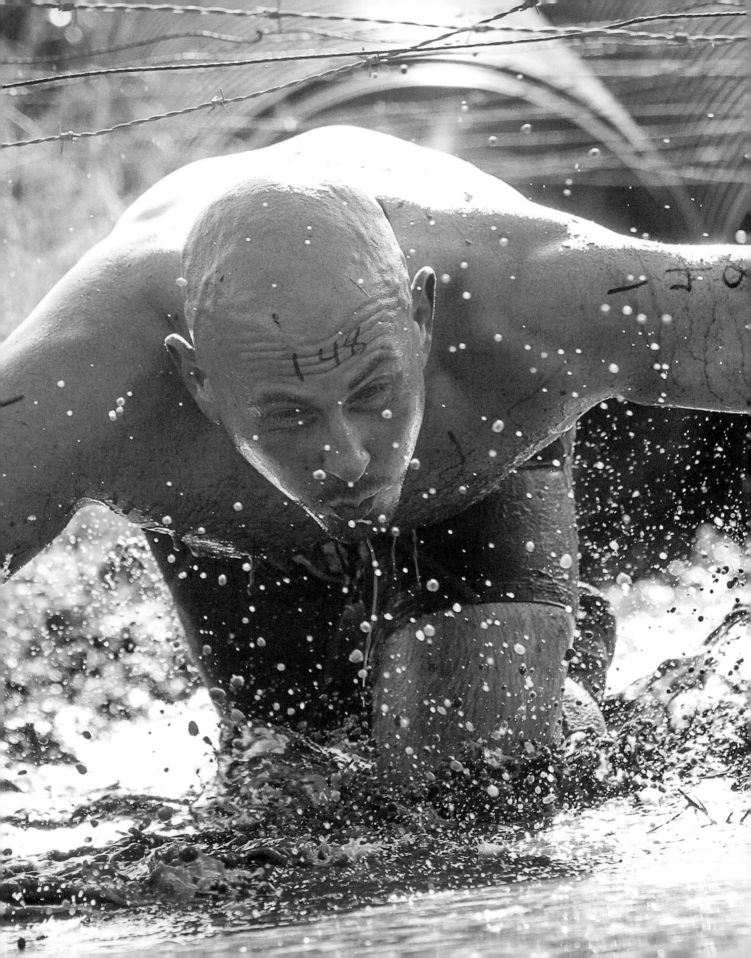

2 THE CURRENT STATE OF OCR

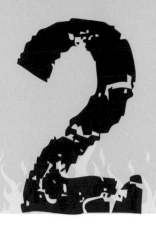

The Big 3 led the explosion in obstacle course racing and mud runs worldwide. In 2010, an estimated twenty events attracted 50,000 participants. In 2011, those numbers grew to seventy events with 250,000 participants. In 2012, the number more than doubled again with 150 events and 1.5 million people signing up to race. In 2013, that number most likely will double again, with more than 300 events and almost 3.5 million entrants.

Hold on though, it's not all Spartan rainbows and Mudder lollipops. With any boom comes several busts. In the recent months before this writing, Hero Rush, Ruckus Race, and the Great American Mud Run recently closed their doors because their goals were bigger than their wallets.

Caught up in the OCR gold rush, new race organizers are planning nationwide tours several months in advance, assuming they'll get thousands of people to turn up, just as they do for every event the Big 3 puts on. Many times, the reality is, they barely break 1,000 participants, or even worse, they only get a few hundred.

Because there are so many races, the smaller events tend to cannibalize one another. Also, what a lot of these smaller companies fail to realize is that while the Big 3 all had small beginnings, they've grown to multimillion-dollar marketing machines. They've spent a pretty penny to attract their now very loyal and ever-growing customer base.

So where are we in terms of the life of OCR? Are we still in infancy? Are we going through growing pains? Everything in this sport happens so fast, it can be tough to tell.

◄ *Don't forget to hold your breath when you are face-deep in mud.*

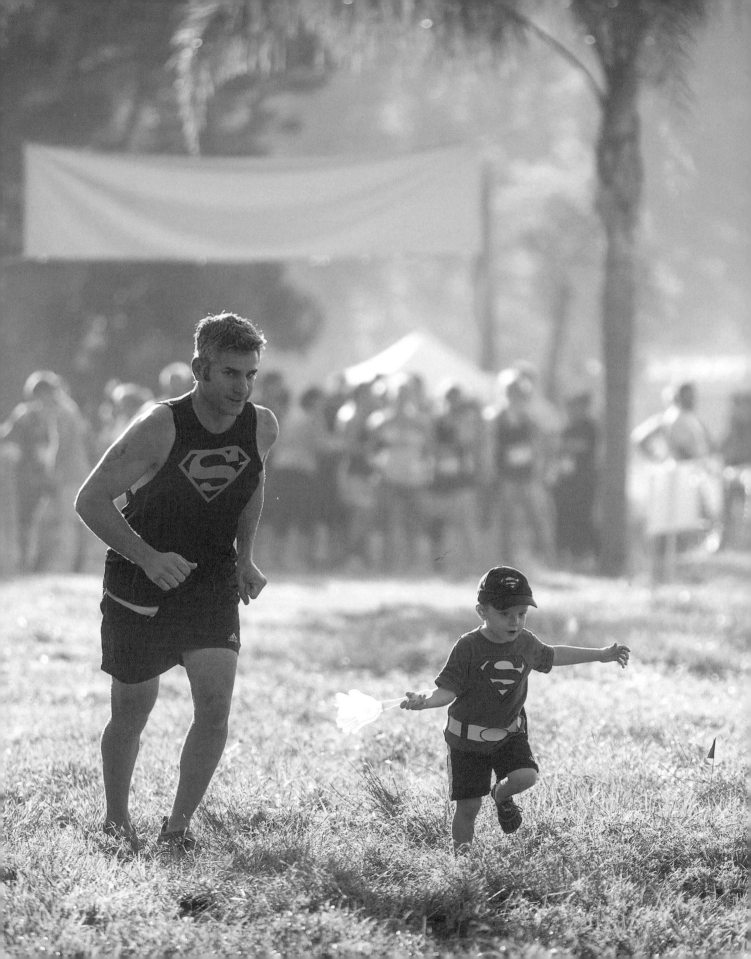

One week, we get news that a new race series with huge payouts is coming. The next week, a well-liked event series goes out of business. In any given week, a familiar OCR athlete goes down with an injury, while a new face pops up no one has heard of, looking prepped to take on all comers.

The most constant state of OCR is change, and that is one of the reasons it is so exciting.

The OCR industry is still so young. We won't have answers to the following questions for a few years.

- Will the Big 3 keep to themselves, or will they start to look at what can be done to organize the sport?

- Will some of the smaller races band together to create some sort of league to compete with the Big 3?

- Will there be a governing body that covers safety and consistency of obstacles?

- Will it all wash away as one giant fad? (Gasp!)

For still other questions, we do have some answers.

FUN AND THEMED RUNS

The incredible growth statistics on page 27 don't include the hundreds of thousands of people who participate in the very popular color, water, foam, or nighttime glow-in-the-dark runs. These races, which often get lumped into obstacle course racing (OCR), are also gaining massive popularity.

These "fun" races offer a chance to sign up with little to no physical fitness of any kind. The events are almost never timed because they are not about being competitive. Instead, they're about getting off the couch and running and/or walking with your spouse, kids, and friends.

These events are far less expensive to produce than obstacle course races. Even though quality fun run events put on a good show, they don't need huge build crews, don't require any obstacles to be built, and don't require dirt to be moved around.

◄ *OCR brings out the whole family.*

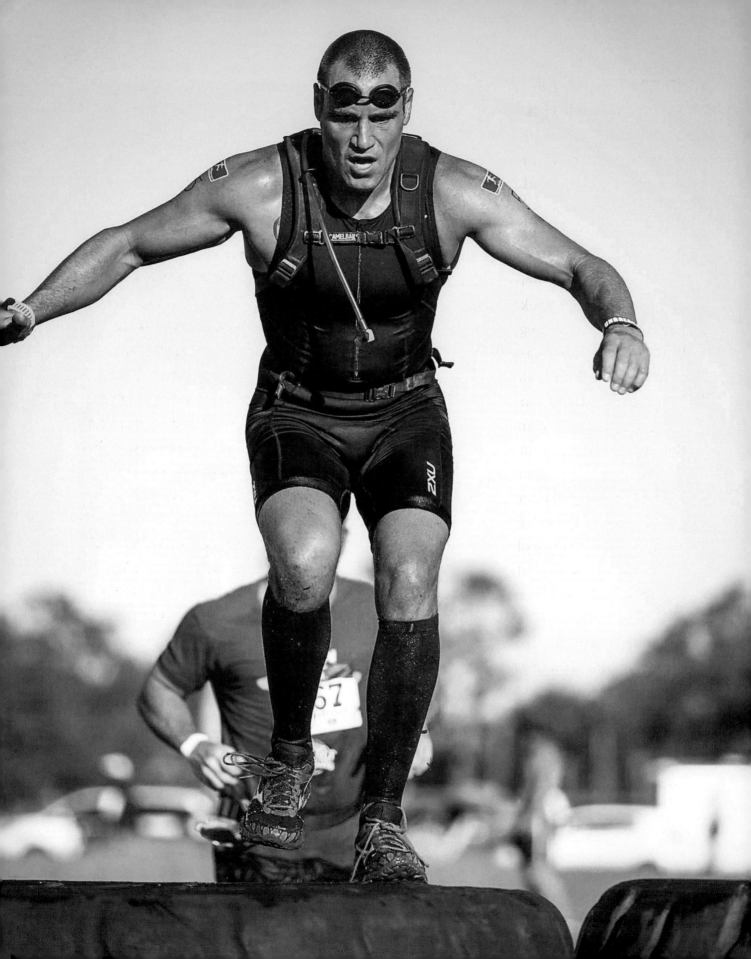

Will There Be More Permanent Races?

One of the shifts we may see in the industry is more permanent race sites. We've already seen successful examples of quality locations putting on high-caliber events. For example, Jonny Simpkins puts on a dozen races a year near Orlando, Florida, at his permanent site for his event series called Rock On Adventures. Camp Rhino, in Las Vegas, has a great training facility, which they are looking to turn into full-on obstacle races. The people over at Dirt Runner, in Illinois, bring in hundreds on any given weekend. Rob Butler and his team at Shale Hill, in Vermont, have an awesome location with some of the most challenging obstacles anywhere. In addition, Butler has already been hired to produce obstacles at another permanent location in upstate New York. What if these permanent sites worked together to somehow form their own race series? They could all save the huge amounts of money that go into "putting a show on the road."

If the permanent race sites in the U.S. don't decide to band together, the successful regional "mom and pop" races might take over by themselves.

Companies such as Mud Endeavor in mid-south Florida, Tuff Scramblers in New England, and Mudathlon in the Midwest, all can have successful events with only 500 to 1,500 participants—although they often bring in many more.

If regional races tried to move their race series all over the country, they could never survive on their numbers. However, keeping it close to home, they can maximize deals with local vendors, save on travel costs, and build relationships with the local race communities that pay back huge dividends. Keeping races local also makes it more likely that the races carve out enough of a name that the traveling races could no longer compete with them, and might stop coming altogether.

In terms of permanent sites in the U.K., there is, first and foremost, Tough Guy. Mr. Mouse adds obstacles every year to his "sufferfest," now with more than 200 obstacles on the 8-mile (12.9 km) course. Another permanent site seeing success is Nuts Challenge, located in Dorking, about an hour south of London. Nuts Challenge has a 4.3-mile (7 km) course with about 100 obstacles per lap. They structure their race to allow more fit/crazy people to do

◄ *Some people transform themselves into beasts through OCR.*

more laps. Newcomers can do 1 lap, while the most fit athletes can sign up for what they call "Tough Nuts," which is 4 laps of the course. This takes even the fittest 4–6 hours to complete. The Commando Challenge is run on an active training center, the Commando Training Centre Royal Marines. Unlike most races, which boast obstacles "inspired by military training," this is the real deal. Athletes run 10 miles (17 km) of an actual obstacle course that aspiring British military complete (within a certain time) to become Royal Marines.

In Australia, Raw Challenge (www .rawchallenge.com.au) on the New South Wales central coast has a permanent course, running two major events each year. Other permanent courses run regular competitive league or themed races, catering to 100 to 300 participants (www.xocr .com.au and www.muddrunners.com.au).

The Emerald Mud Run, in Central Queensland, attracts more than 1,500 to a small town of only 13,000 people. That's a huge turnout when more than 10 percent of the town is attending (www.mudrun emerald.com.au)! You can find a mud run in northern Tasmania twice a year (www .tasmudrun.com.au) and Mud Sweat and Beers (www.mudsweatandbeers.com.au) and Blood Sweat and Fears (www .bloodsweatandfears.com.au) in Wagga

and Darwin respectively. All three are in townships of less than 150,000 people, yet are back for their second showing in 2014.

Will OCR Go Mainstream?

The biggest question everyone in OCR wants answered is this: Can the sport cross over into the mainstream? For this to happen, larger dollars need to be involved. In 2013, those dollars started coming, but not enough to put OCR in front of the average person. Reebok made a deal with Spartan for an undisclosed sum. But other than renaming the race itself and putting the Reebok name on a few obstacles, not much changed.

Wheaties put a photo of Tough Mudder's Everest obstacle on boxes this year. But will that turn people on to obstacle course racing?

Along with attracting large sponsors, getting the sport on television is the other obvious key to getting OCR in front of the most eyeballs. One race series, Hard Charge, has already begun televising taped races in several markets across the United States.

In December 2013, Spartan Race aired its largest race of the year, in Vermont, for the NBC Sports Network.

Although there's some positive momentum going on, some things are happening that may hurt the sport in the

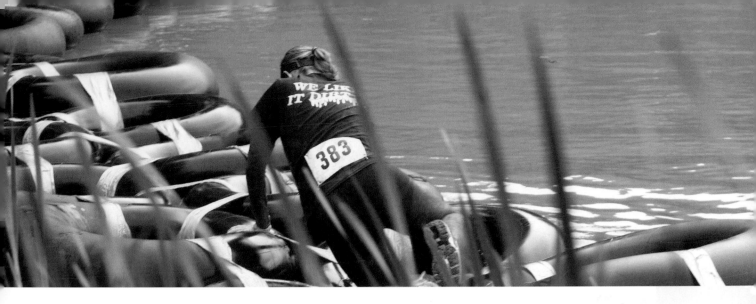

▲ *Do you think one day you'll see your coworker complete an obstacle like this?*

long term. Fly-by-night companies are launching Facebook pages and websites promising a good time. Then, through either poor event management or flat-out thievery, they don't deliver on what they promise. After the event, attendees post on Facebook or through the OCR grapevine that a race had minimal and/or poorly constructed obstacles, no beer or food as promised, ran out of medals, or ran out of water. The list of problems goes on and on.

Other races are cancelled or postponed before they even start due to low registration numbers. Again, it could have been because of a poor marketing plan, or someone who just set out to rip people off.

This may convince racers to stay home and to never again register for another race—other than their local 5k or marathon. The other option is that maybe only the Big 3 will survive because people won't risk their dollars on any unknown entities.

As it stands now, obstacle course racing is still growing in overall participation. That's the good—no, *great*—news for you who have chosen to read this book.

If you haven't signed up for a race yet, the next three chapters are going to be extremely helpful. I am going to help you choose your first race, find or start an OCR group in your area, and, with the help of my friend Muddy Mommy, give you a general overview on preparing you for your first race.

The remaining chapters will be for the newbie and OCR veteran alike as we talk to experts on how to eat, train, and conquer obstacles.

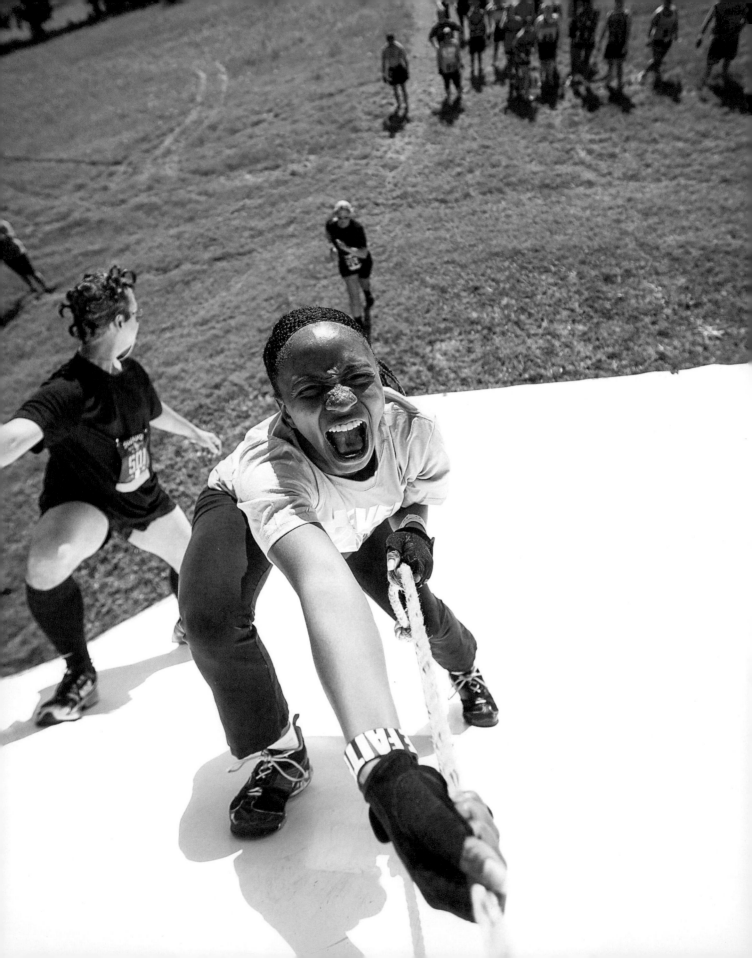

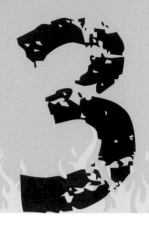

3 GETTING READY FOR YOUR FIRST RACE

❦ Featuring Holly Joy Berkey, a.k.a. Muddy Mommy

Subsequent chapters in this book will go into great detail on how to train and prepare for obstacle course races. Those chapters will talk about nutrition, training for specific obstacles, and lots of various tips and tricks. In the meantime, I want to give a general overview on how you might approach your first race, having previously done little or no training.

❦ ❦ ❦

Two years ago, I had never run a race, never pinned a numbered bib to my shirt, and never fastened a chip timer to my shoe. I had no clue how to select the right shoe for my stride, calculate my pace, or properly train for a race. I wasn't a runner, much less a runner who trained to run races. Running was a mystery to me, and I lived my life blissfully unaware that the quickly growing sport of obstacle course racing would soon become a great passion of mine.

Fast forward to today. After making the decision to take an active interest in my health, I shed fifty pounds, I run almost daily, and I *love* to race! I've become the obstacle racer I never thought possible, and I'm still amazed by how much in my life has drastically changed. I feel like a different person! Had you told me two years ago that my favorite way to spend a Saturday would be to get up early and drive a couple of hours to a tiny town in the middle of nowhere to run races through the mud, I probably would have thought you were a crazy person.

Yet, here I am.

◀ *This can be you in no time!*

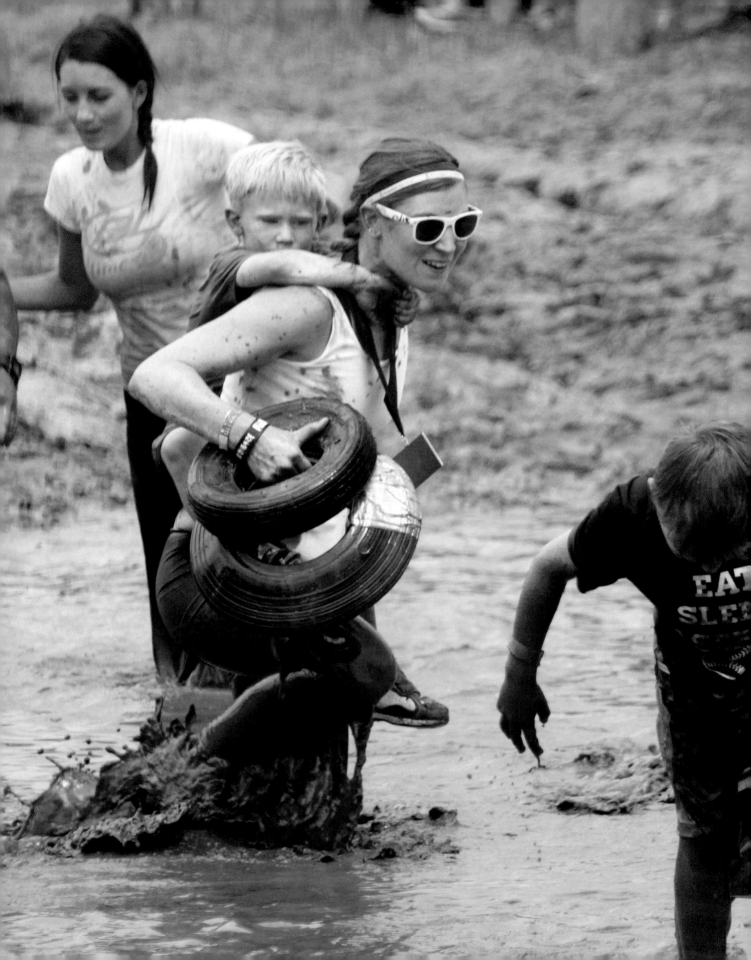

Why am I telling you this? Well, my point is this: Everyone has to start somewhere. The majority of people have not been athletes their entire lives, but that doesn't mean that we cannot make a change in our adult lives to positively impact our health. We have to make a conscious choice to change. We can choose to continue living a life that is sedentary and apathetic, or we can begin working toward a healthier, happier existence by taking an active interest in our own health and well-being.

I had my realization in March 2011. At 193 pounds (88 kg) and barely able to squeeze into a size 12, I was sick of feeling fat, hating how I looked, and being embarrassed of myself. I didn't feel good about myself, and it directly affected how I enjoyed my daily life. I finally decided that just because I was a mom, worked full time, and was a busy person that didn't mean that I should give up on having a body that I was proud of. I began gradually changing my lifestyle.

Slowly but surely, I shed pounds through proper diet and exercise. And then, going against my own reservations, I ran my first mud run. My life changed forever.

Since December 2012, I've completed nineteen obstacle races. People who are contemplating running their first races regularly ask me how to properly train for such an event. I believe that a few key items are perfect advice for anyone on the fence about trying an obstacle race.

For starters, I like to remind people that obstacle course racing is physically challenging, and it's also mentally chal-

"Going against my own reservations, I ran my first mud run. My life changed forever."

lenging. It seems to me that the majority of people who are longing to experience an obstacle race, but have yet to actually pull the trigger and sign up, seem to be held back by one main factor: their own self-doubts. People give me all kinds of excuses for why they have yet to give an obstacle race a try, such as, "I'm afraid I can't complete the obstacles," "I'm not a runner," "I'll probably hurt myself," and "I'm not a strong swimmer."

◄ *Muddy Mommy changed her whole life through obstacle racing.*

My Simple Advice

To people getting started with OCR, I have three pieces of advice.

STOP SELLING YOURSELF SHORT! You *can* do it! You can do anything you put your mind to, so why not take on a new endeavor and try an event that will challenge you while getting you out of your comfort zone? We humans are extremely resilient, and we've been accomplishing astounding feats for centuries. You're no different, and the only reason you haven't accomplished this yet is simply because you haven't allowed yourself to. Put aside your fear, worry, and self-deprecating attitude, and get out and try it! You'll probably have a fantastic time proving yourself wrong. You'll need to prepare your mind for the

> "Humans are extremely resilient, and we've been accomplishing astounding feats for centuries."

task of training, of showing up to the race, and then of completing the race when you reach a point where you do not feel like you can continue. But the second you cross that finish line, you'll gain a pride in yourself that no one can take away. So please, repeat this over and over until your brain finally accepts it, "Yes, I can do it."

YOU HAVE TO REGISTER FOR A RACE TO RUN IT. The sooner you register, the sooner you and your butt have "signed on the dotted line." Your brain and body will change by committing to going. You show this commitment by signing up.

Another chapter in this book will address how to choose that first race to sign up for. Skip ahead to that chapter if you like, and then come back here.

Here's my own simple advice for choosing a race. If you have OCR friends who already participate in races, find out which one they are doing next, and sign up. If you're the first person you know to try an OCR, look online for races near you, pick one, and plunk that credit card down.

YOU MUST PREPARE. Although I encourage every person—of any shape or size—to try an obstacle course race if he/she are intrigued by the sport, if you want to actually *enjoy* the entire race experience, you really do need to prepare for it. That's not to say you won't love a certain obstacle, cherish crossing the finish line and receiving your medal, or savor that post-race beer. But if you don't actually do some race preparation, there are also some parts of the race that you may actually hate—immensely. The running, climbing, crawling, and the burpee

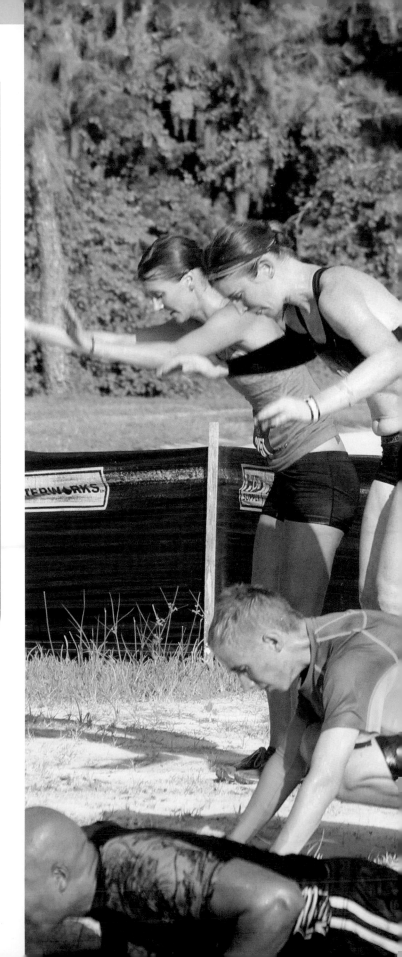

BURPEES

Certain races have penalties for not completing certain obstacles. Burpees are one of the most popular penalties instituted at these competitive obstacle races. Spartan Race was the first to institute burpees, and many races have followed suit. Proper form is a variable that changes among the various race series. Here is the eight-count burpee that Spartan insists upon for their races.

1. Start from a standing position.
2. Drop to a squat with your hands on the ground.
3. Extend your legs back so you are in a plank position.
4. Go down into a pushup.
5. Come back up from the pushup.
6. Return your feet to a squat position.
7. Stand back up.
8. Jump up, having your feet leave the ground. (Some people clap at this point.)

penalties—at some events they're inevitable, even for the most seasoned athlete! Although some participants decide to spend their pre-race days doing no exercise whatsoever, I'd bet money that those are also the racers who are the most

▶ *You may skip an obstacle but be ready to do burpees at some events.*

self-loathing for a few days post-race, as they nurse their battered and bruised bodies that aren't used to any sort of physical activity.

Obstacle course races are a challenge; they're supposed to be. If they weren't, they wouldn't have the widespread appeal that they have today. There seems to be a curiosity ingrained in each of us that makes us seek out new challenges, that craves excitement, and that gets a thrill when we're pushed to our limits and live to tell about it. We want to do things that make us proud of ourselves. We want the bragging rights to say, "I accomplished this!" But succeeding at any challenge takes preparation. Skipping that important part sets you up for potential failure and disappointment.

Granted, to prepare for a race, you don't need to drop everything and dig yourself into hours of training each day. That's the perfect way to set yourself up for failure because you burn out within a matter of weeks—or days!—and give up. Start slowly: Go for a run with friends, join a gym, or sign up for a boot camp, spinning, or Zumba class. Find something that interests you! Just don't do *nothing*.

Think of it like this: It's not smart to skip studying before a big exam, right? Just like you need to exercise your brain before testing it, you need to exercise your body to prepare it for several miles of running and climbing over obstacles. Properly preparing will help you feel happier and healthier, you'll gain confidence in your ability to complete the race, and you'll be so proud of your accomplishment when you cross the finish line.

My Training Recommendations

So how do I do this, you ask? There's no set formula for how to train for obstacle course racing, but my recommendation to all new racers is to begin mixing in cardio/endurance workout with some strength training. Obstacle course racing is unique because it requires the stamina to run or walk several miles, and also the strength to complete obstacles that require a fair amount of upper body and core strength. If you only run to prepare, or if you only lift weights, you may find that you do not feel adequately prepared for a great deal of what the race will require of you.

▶ *Stretching pre- and post-race can be crucial.*

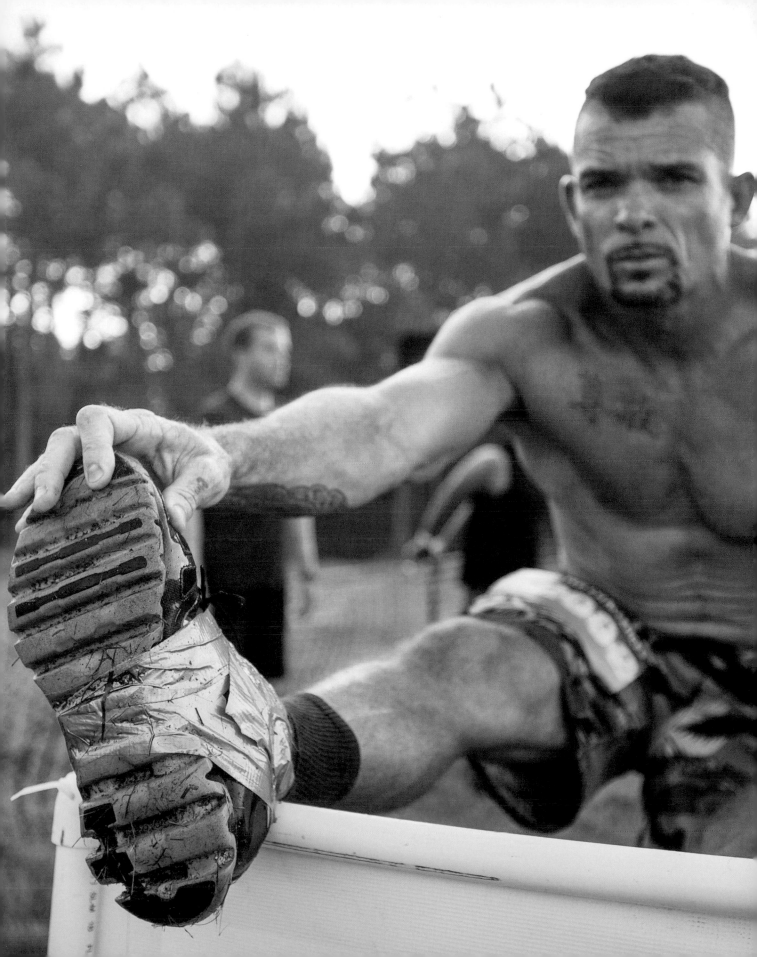

I say this especially to females, who tend to lack in upper body strength. When I completed the monkey bars obstacle in a race for the first time, I got so excited that I almost hugged the complete stranger next to me! I was elated that I had finally trained well enough to complete an obstacle that, in prior races, I hadn't been able to finish.

Many obstacle course races include walls to scale, ropes to climb, sandbags to carry, monkey bars to traverse, buckets to lift, and many other upper-body strength challenges. Weight training, or even body-weight exercises such as planks and push-ups, are a huge help to gain upper-body strength.

Also, to prepare for an OCR, you need to run, if only a little. It's been a while since I can remember getting winded after a ¼-mile (0.4 km) run, but I remember that it's no fun to be gassed out and feel like you have nothing left in you to give when you still have miles to go. Running combined with some strength training will get you a step closer to a finish you are proud of, and you'll love the physical results you see as well! Try to shoot for two or three days of running per week, and work in weight training, boot camp,

or some sort of strength-training exercises on the alternating days. Trust me, it'll make a difference.

I've participated in quite a few mud runs thus far in my short career of racing, and I hope to continue running them for as long as the sport is around. One of my favorite things about obstacle course races is that at any event, you'll see every type of physique imaginable. You'll encounter people who are elite athletes, as well as those who are considered morbidly obese, but who have finally decided to make a positive step toward a healthy lifestyle. All are welcome in this sport, no one is left out, and all join in the fun.

"At any event, you'll see every type of physique imaginable."

Another great thing about obstacle course racing is that you can run the events seriously to feed your competitive spirit, or you can walk the entire course if you so choose. Most participants choose to embark with a group of close friends, encouraging and helping each other along the way, completing the course as a team. To me, camaraderie and teamwork are

▶ *Some obstacles can not be trained for.*

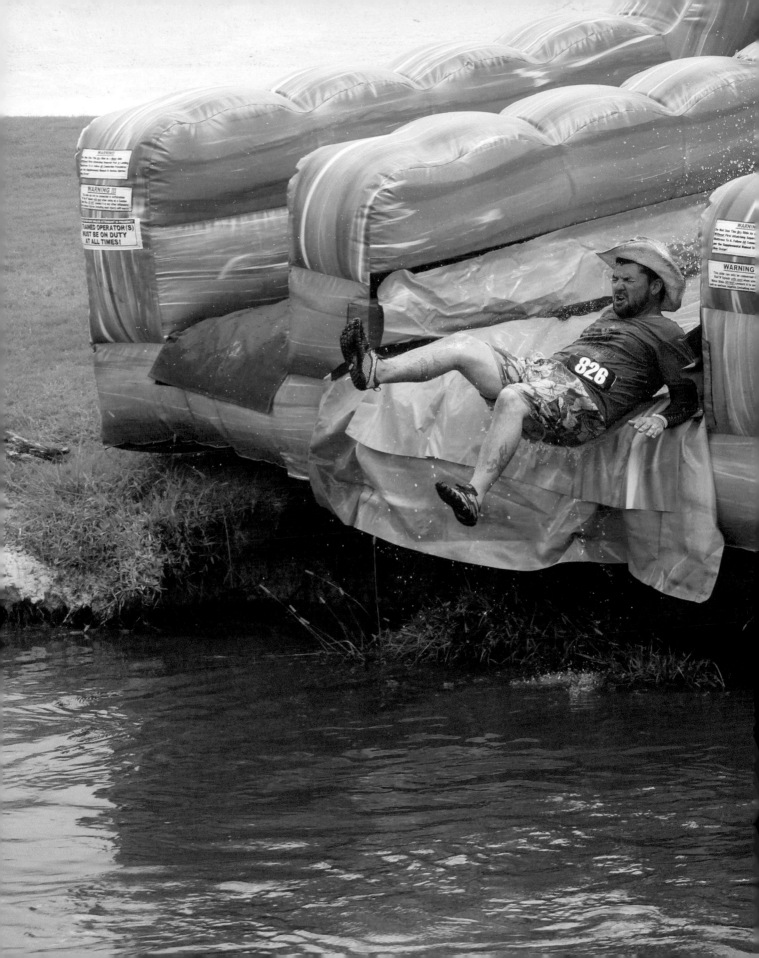

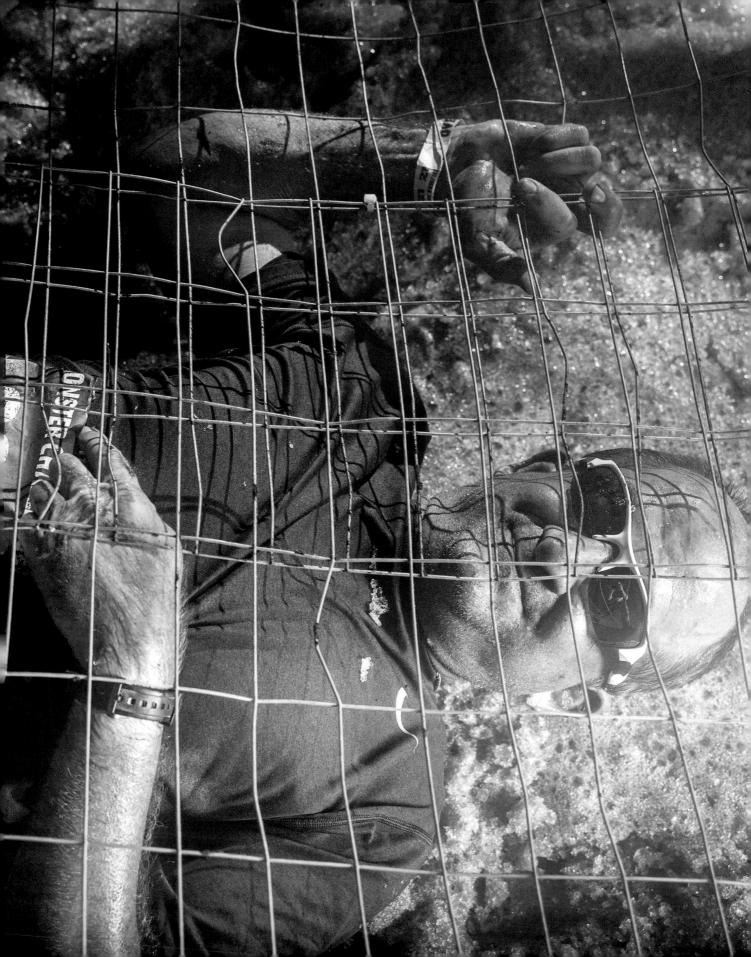

really what obstacle racing is all about. This type of event is not the "every person for themselves" kind of sport. Rather, OCR is built to bring people together in a world that has become so very disconnected and individualistic.

Now it's time to stop worrying, stop doubting yourself, and sign up for a race. Train a little, or a lot, find some friends who will join you, and enjoy your experience. Be proud of yourself as you push past your fears and conquer each obstacle as it comes. When you finish—and you *will* finish—celebrate your accomplishment! Enjoy your well-earned medal, your delicious free beer, and the elated feeling that you have just completed something that you were recently too intimidated to even try.

I encourage you to take this one step further, and tell the world. Post pictures of yourself caked in mud, hands raised, with a huge smile on your face. Let the world know you did something you were unsure about just a few weeks before. You never know, your photo may inspire someone else to do the same.

DOWN AND DIRTY TAKEAWAYS

- **Sign up.** Pull out your credit card and sign up for a race. Don't wait until you are "ready."
- **Prepare for greater enjoyment.** People of any fitness level can enjoy obstacle racing, but preparing more can mean *lots* more fun.
- **Find your own path.** There's no set training formula. Find the form of training that works for you.
- **Enjoy the spoils.** When the race is over, enjoy that beer, wear that medal, and post pictures like crazy. You earned it.

Holly Joy Berkey turned herself from couch potato to OCR fanatic in a relatively short time, so much so that now she is known as "Muddy Mommy." Holly discovered her love of running in 2011, after making the choice to pursue a healthier lifestyle. Through exercise and improving her diet, she lost 50 pounds (22.7 kg)—all while balancing the daily challenges of family and career. She documents her experiences in running, training, and racing on her blog www.muddymommy.com.

◄ *You may see everything through new glasses after a few events.*

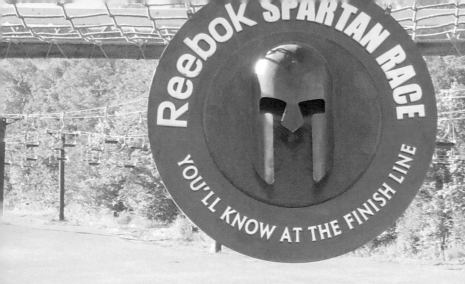

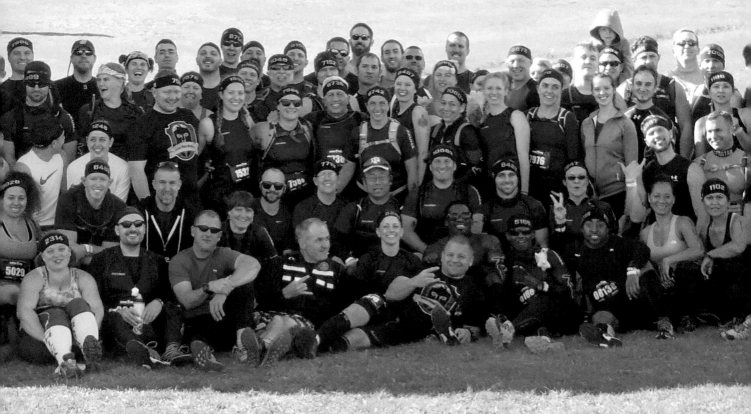

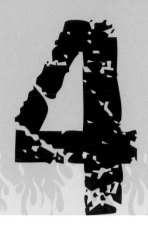

FINDING OR STARTING AN OCR GROUP

☙ Featuring Paul Jones of the New England Spahtens

Paul Jones calls himself the "Idea Wrangler" at the New England Spahtens. He's one of the founders of the group, and he's a very proactive leader. I asked him to contribute to this chapter because the Spahtens are a great example of what being part of an OCR community does for so many people.

☙ ☙ ☙

When I was asked to contribute to this book, I thought, "There really is no better way to respond than to ask the New England Spahtens themselves." So I did.

You'll find quotes from active members of this successful community throughout this chapter. For example:

"Being a part of this team has reminded me that I'm strong . . . and even when I don't believe it, someone else around me believes it extra hard for me. And it has given me the incredible gift of being a small part of great people doing epic stuff—all the way from our Winter Death Race champions, to people hitting the podium, to someone finishing their first race—or even just signing up for it."
—*Jennifer, Spahtens team member*

"Oh jeez, how do I count the ways? Well, I have no family in this state, so this team is pretty much my family. So many of you have encouraged me and been there for me in so many ways. For example, just at the Superhero Scramble, Dennis patched me up, Paul

◀ *The New England Spahtens is of one of the largest and most successful OCR groups in the country.*

let me use his headlamp for a whim decision in the night heat, Bobby held me up on the mountain when my blood sugar plummeted, Tom held me up when I got off the mountain. I mean, good lawd, I don't believe there is a way to describe the awesomeness of this team. I've been pushed way beyond my comfort zone and found I am so much more capable than I believed. Thanks so much, y'all."

—*Marcie, Spahtens team member*

My Story

Personally, I found obstacle course racing "early," running the second-ever Spartan Race in 2010 with a few of my gym buddies. We also ran Rugged Maniac and Ruckus in the same year. In 2011, life got in the way, and my little team went off to do their own thing. But I was hooked.

I ran several races in 2011, and by 2012, I was looking for more. Unfortunately, I had no one to run with. My gym mates, other friends, and even my neighbors were all done with racing, and I was left with the prospect of signing up for a race solo. So I got involved with the Spartan Race Street Team, and then by extension, the MA (Massachusetts) Spartans.

Initially, the MA Spartans and their slightly more southern counterparts, the RI (Rhode Island) Spartans, were two very separate groups whose only real priority was the Spartan Race series. Members came from the Spartan Race Street Team, and the main focus was on how they could support and promote the Spartan Race events. A random meeting of minds at the MA Spartan Sprint race in August 2012 brought about a very quick merger of the two groups on Facebook, and the New England Spahtens was born.

"I've been pushed way beyond my comfort zone and found I am so much more capable than I believed."

Building a Team

I was lucky enough to be chosen to be part of the group administrator, initially just to police for spammers. But it turned into a catalyst for something bigger—and much better. Humble beginnings.

We had a little Facebook group, but we had no website, Twitter account, or even Facebook page. We were just a group of around a hundred people who shared a common interest. We started to talk about creating a logo, and a pretty quick vote in the group settled on the merger of the helmet and anchor to represent our strength and our New England roots.

Next we started a website, where I blogged about anything and everything OCR-related. Initially, the focus was content. We shared discount codes for upcoming races and gear, race experiences, and stories.

Once the blogging took hold, two things really helped set us apart from "just another race team."

OUR BRAND. The first thing that sets us apart is our brand. We were fortunate enough to have a designer in the team who made our amazing helmet-and-anchor logo. The helmet was a nod to the MA Spartans group, and the anchor was in homage to the RI Spartans. We brought in the rest of New England, and our focus and identity was born. This design ended up going on our amazing drill shirts, which are the highly technical, fitted shirts you see our members wear in races. Those shirts aren't cheap, but buying a shirt gives our members something more than just a cool piece of clothing. It gives them an identity. Anywhere they wear their drill shirts, they're recognized as part of something bigger than being just "another guy at a race."

▶ *OCR is in many ways about teamwork.*

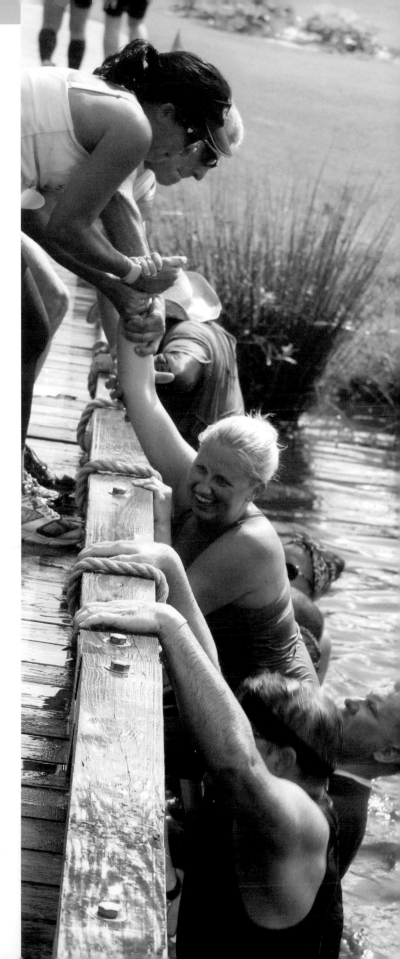

OUR FOCUS. The second thing that sets us apart from being "just another race team" is our focus. I started reaching out to race directors and bluntly asking them to provide a discount code. Don't ask, don't get, right? Some race directors declined, but others obliged. Some were shocked by my request, but others seemed excited by the chance to work with our new race community. Smart race directors gave us discounts that would encourage people to join in, and we were excited to promote 10 percent, 20 percent, or higher discounts. Some race directors were a little shortsighted and found themselves missing out.

When I talked to race directors, the image I tried to convey was that we are a highly organized, driven team with a very clear focus, and that we wanted to participate in and promote obstacle course racing in the New England region. That's it. Clear, easy to digest. Some race communities try for national or even global status, with differing levels of success, but our regional focus made us successful quickly.

And we grew. Every race we attended, we wore our drill shirts proudly. We organized using Facebook events in our group. We helped other racers on the course, and we talked to them in the festival areas. Mondays and Tuesdays after races, people joined our Facebook community in droves, after they got back to work and remembered "the guys in the blue shirts with the funny name."

As our group grew in membership, we also grew in scope. What was initially just a way to enjoy obstacle course racing with our buddies became more. People joined from all over the New England region, and we started meeting to train in those unique and weird ways we train for obstacle course races. People started meeting to hike mountains or carry logs. People started hosting get-togethers in their yards, and we spent mornings climbing ropes, walls, and rucking (doing runs and workouts carrying some form of weighted ruck), and then we kicked back with a beer and barbecue.

> "People started hosting get-togethers in their yards, and we spent mornings climbing ropes, walls, and rucking."

Friendships started to form. We found that we were interested in this sport of OCR, and also that we liked each other.

▶ *Mudrunfun lives up to their name. Here they carry their team flag through an entire course.*

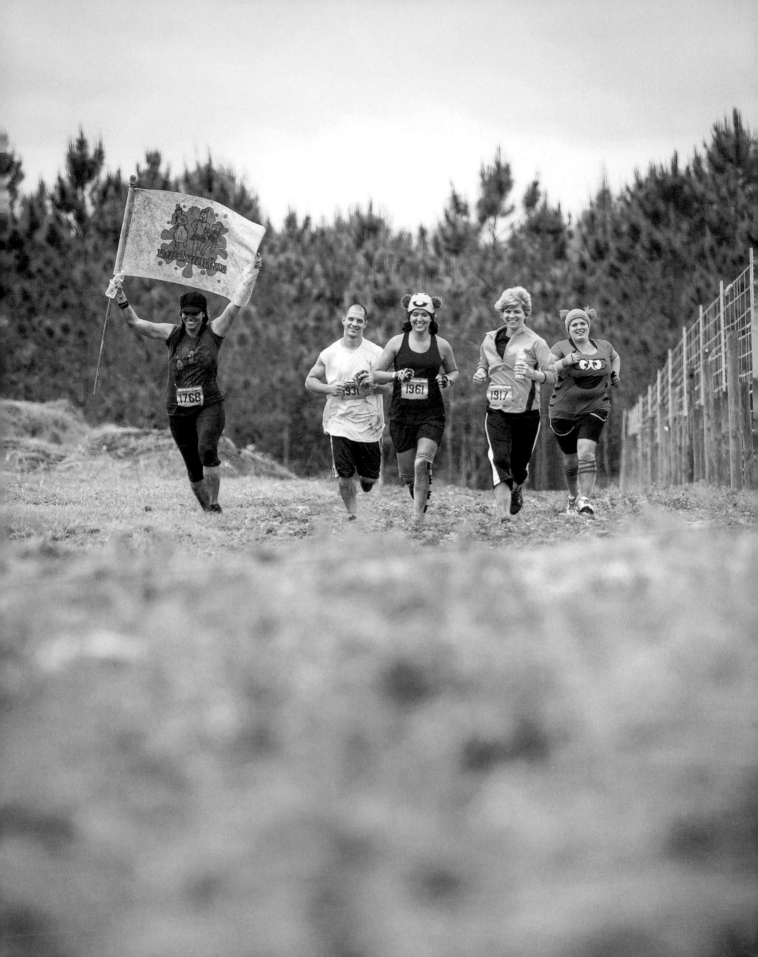

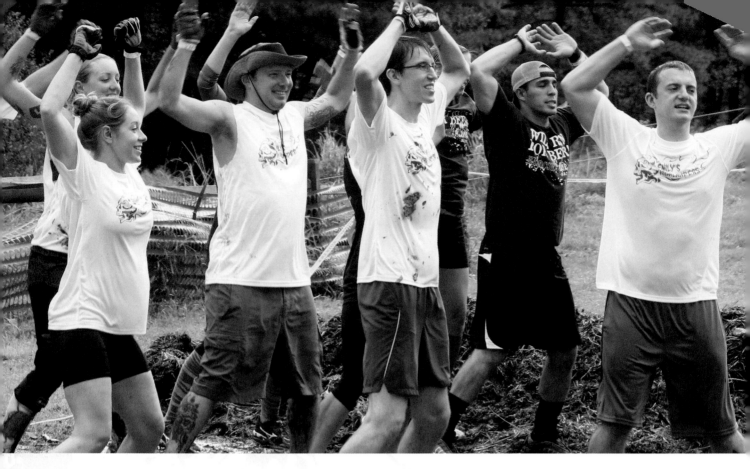

▲ *Suffering through exercises can be more fun with friends.*

As new people joined, they were quickly absorbed into this all-inclusive community of folks whose only common interest—at least on the surface—was racing in the mud and climbing over things.

I can remember spending Cyber Monday, 2012, at my desk. From the moment I woke up to the moment I went back to sleep, I did very little other than share race information and race gear deals. The smart and organized races made sure they had deals ready to go, and it was a huge task to keep up with them. Many of us nearly filled our race calendars on that one day alone.

The stories of how our team and community had affected people began pouring in.

"Before I came aboard, I thought I was in good shape. I always work out. Now that I'm part of this group, I am becoming different. I am regularly doing things that I would have never done before. I am growing and improving. What I once thought was not possible is now becoming routine. Do not accept your limits!"

—*Robert, Spahtens team member*

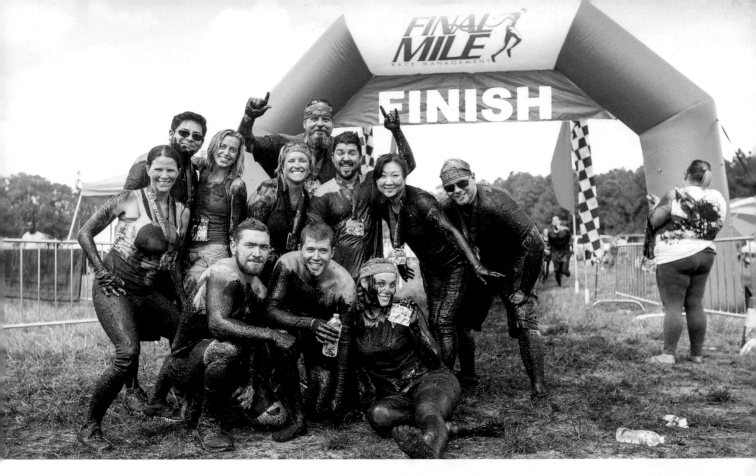

▲ *Posing together for epic photo-ops is more fun as a group, too.*

"Sandy Rhee (unknowingly even to her) brainwashed me with her positive attitude. As for the rest of you Spahtens, well, you are an infectious bunch of fun folks who have unleashed a wanna-be-better streak in me."
—*Jeanine, Spahtens team member*

"Do not accept your limits!"

We grew. We now had Facebook communities dedicated to training, a Facebook page, and a Twitter account. Our blog was getting hundreds of unique hits a day, and this was only a few months into our life. The growth of the team was dramatic, and that rosy view I had initially projected to race directors was becoming a reality. We were hitting hundreds of members, and we were well organized.

In December 2012, I got a message from a venue owner. He told me that he had built the very best fixed obstacle course in the country, and he was holding an endurance race in the middle of January. The race would consist of racers running as many laps as possible in eight hours. In Vermont. In the snow. The owner planned

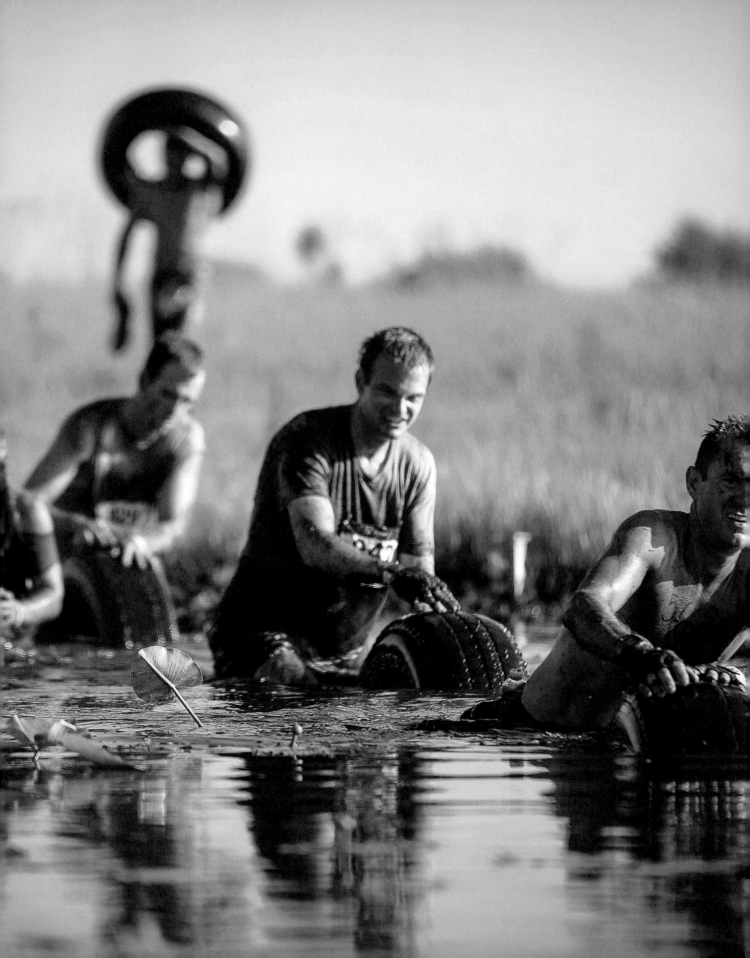

to cater all day, too—with a never-ending supply of bacon.

It sounded almost ludicrous. I'd never heard of him, his venue, or his race. When I reached out to some of my new race director contacts, even one who grew up in the next town, they hadn't heard of him either. After one race director checked around for two weeks, he came back with the simple message that yes, Rob Butler of Shale Hill Adventure Farms is legit. Done. Sold. We were in. We brought more than a dozen people to that first event—the 2012 Polar Bear Challenge—taking the biggest team. That same day, we also brought the biggest team of more than thirty people to a second obstacle course race, the Blizzard Blast.

> "Never in my wildest dreams did I think this small obstacle course race support group we started back in the day could and would become a contending, full-on racing team. Not just elites, but supportive enthusiasts willing to help each other, and be there for newcomers. Spahtens, to me, embody what it truly means to be a team. No one is left behind, and no one is put on a pedestal. We all matter!"
> —*Nate, Spahtens team member*

At this point, we had a good framework in place, with the following tools available to our community.

- **A FACEBOOK GROUP FOR THE MAIN COMMUNITY CHATTER:** Facebook is an easy, handy place for people to chat and discuss things related to obstacle course racing.

- **A FACEBOOK PAGE:** We use it to broadcast industry information, such as local race price changes.

- **A WEBSITE:** Over time, it's grown from a simple blog full of our random opinions and race reviews into a full website, including featured reviews, community sources reviews, expert opinions, motivational posts, a store, training programs, featured athlete profiles, and recipes. If someone asked for it, we tried to find a way to provide it.

- **TEAM GEAR:** At every race, we were recognized, and as the races passed, we got more and more familiar with the race scene. This was in no small part due to our shirts. Made by UK Rugby supplier Akuma, our drill shirts are super high-quality, 100 percent printed compression tops. Customized

◄ *On a hot day, you appreciate the little things, like wading across a cool pond.*

with the racer's nickname and absolutely badass, the more people who started wearing these drill shirts, the more of a uniform it became. We have since expanded into other team gear, but the drill shirts remain a favorite with the group. They really stand out when other local teams are still writing on cheap cotton T-shirts with permanent markers. Our uniform makes a massive difference in how seriously we're taken.

Growing a Team

The more recognition we got, the more people would look us up after seeing us at a race. It became common for us to run at a race, and then spend the next few days approving people into our Facebook group, picking up a dozen, twenty, or more new members after each race.

Like any community, no matter how big you become, there is always going to be a core group of folks who are more active than the others. We've been lucky that our core groups of people have formed firm friendships, sometimes relationships beyond that, and for the most part are a friendly, rowdy bunch who love being active, enjoy the competition of race day, and

come to many events. As the team grows, this central core group is also expanding, with very few personality conflicts.

The year 2012 moved along pretty quickly. Members of our community won the Spartan Winter Death Race, which is an ultra-endurance event in Vermont, in the dead of winter. After multiple days and nights in the snow, with our entire Facebook community hanging onto every single update, Josh Grant and Nele Schulze crossed the closest thing the Death Race has to a finish line in first place for men and women. We took biggest team awards at MuckFest MS, Foam Fest, Ruckus, Superhero Scramble (the biggest team they had ever had, with more than one hundred participants wearing Batman character costumes!), a Superhero Scramble in another state, Civilian Military Combine, and a few local races. After each race, new folks would come knocking on our Facebook "doors" on Monday, looking for information on how they could join this crazy group of people in their awesome shirts and asking how they could get more involved.

We trained together at Harvard Stadium, the Stone Tower, and up in

▶ *No one is getting over this wall without a team.*

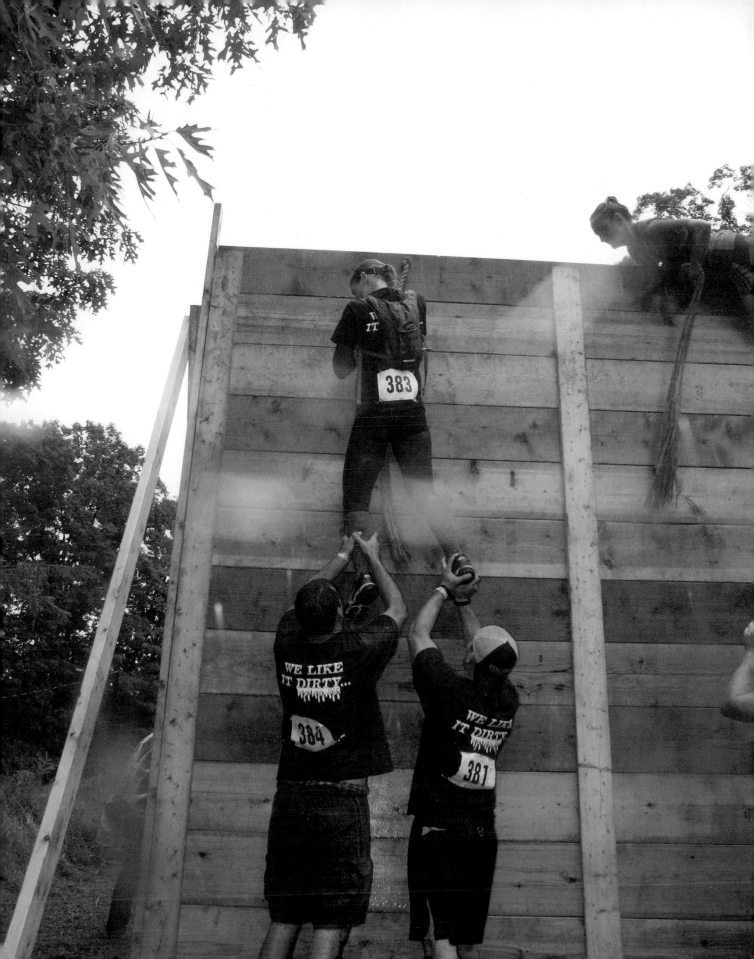

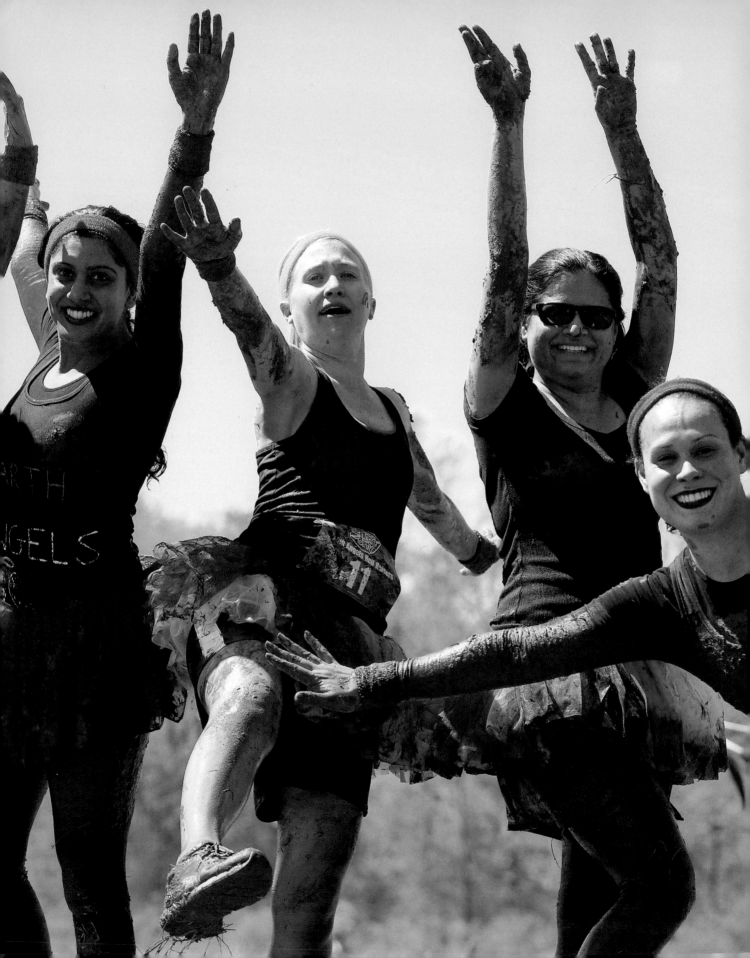

the Granite State. We did CrossFit workouts together at Reebok CrossFit One and hiked mountains together. We spent weekends racing together.

Importantly, we also let our hair down and socialized together. We let our spouses meet the newfound friends who had become such big parts of our lives. We also let our kids play (our little Spahtkins), and we engaged each other in a social setting that didn't involve Spandex and compression gear.

"I was that quiet and shy little fat girl kids picked last in school. I was never really good at sports or very outgoing. I found myself and then lost myself again. Life has been hard for me, and it still is at times. One day, my cousin decided to get a bunch of people into a race (Warrior Dash). I was bit by a mudbug. And then somehow along the way, I met some Spahtens who made me believe in myself again. Who made me see it was okay not to be the fastest or the strongest. Because as long as I was out there, trying, I was successful. I was something, somebody. And somewhere in all that mud, in all the bruises, cuts, pain, smiles, and laughter, I not only found myself again, I found a family—people who encourage me, support me, and I know are there for me! And I hope they know that I would do anything for them!"
—*Denise, Spahtens team member*

The Summer Death Race came around—right in our backyard. We had more people attending from the community than pretty much any other community. We had more people volunteering, too. After three days of racing, in brutal conditions, five people from our community came home with the trophy: finishers' skulls. We threw them a party, and the entire community was caught up, once again, in the circus that was the Death Race.

Closing in on our one-year anniversary event, the MA Spartan Race, we broke the 1,000 member milestone in our group. We already knew we were going to be biggest team at the race. In the end, we had more than 270 registrations for the Saturday race, and fifty-four for the Sunday race, which unofficially made us the biggest team the MA Spartan has ever seen.

The logistics behind that were crazy. To save some sanity, I created a series

◄ *Racers will often wear costumes or team uniforms—but be prepared, they might get ruined.*

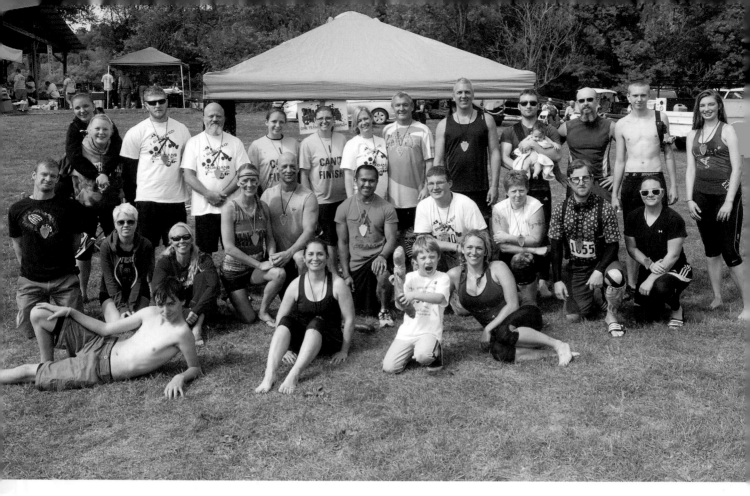

▲ *The Crazy Muddy Muckers are another great OCR group. See Appendix A on page 214 to find a group like this near you.*

of blog posts to answer all the common questions new folks would be asking. Many of those people were being ripped off of the couch for their first event, in true Spartan style. The blog posts answered questions about what to wear, what to pack, and what to expect, including silly little tips that made all the difference on race day, such as not to shave the day before and not to wear cotton undies. The blogs were a lifesaver, both for me as an admin, and for the Spartan crew that was helping me get everyone's questions answered in a timely manner.

Today, our Facebook group has more than 1,100 members, and our core group is growing. More and more new members are finding that being a part of the core group is fun. It's friendly, and it pushes you to be better and stay active.

Race directors are seeing that we have a community with every level of athlete in it—from weekend warriors to obstacle course race experts. We're talking with our members in wider capacities than ever before. In addition to bringing large numbers of people to events, we also consult, advise, and recommend. We have

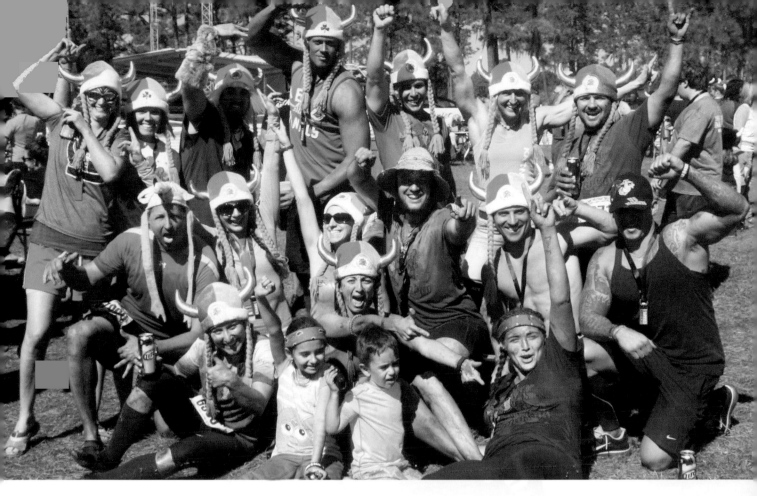

▲ *This is Mud Run Fun from Florida. They usually live up to their name.*

a fully stocked store, including stickers, shirts, decals, iPhone cases, and more. Our members are excited at the chance to represent the team and the community.

"I ran my first official 5k in January, and, because of you guys, completed my first half [marathon] four months later. Even when I'm convinced I can't do something, there are so many more of you who are convinced I can. The encouragement and faith in each other are endless, and when I need a swift kick to get my ass in gear, there's someone more than happy to provide that as well. Never done a Spartan race? Oh, just drink some more Kool-Aid and complete your trifecta. You guys are amazing and never fail to inspire me."
—*Heather, Spahtens team member*

Obstacle course racing as a sport is huge, but it would be boring to me if not for the community it's forged. The friends I've made in the New England Spahtens are a huge, important factor in my life, and I see my role as an administrator to make the Spahtens a huge, reward-ing, and important part of their lives. Everything I've done to date has been with this goal in mind: making the team a better part of people's lives.

If you love this sport, I highly recom-mend joining your own regional communi-ty group. It will only bring you good things.

❧ ❧ ❧

❧ A word from the author:

I trust what Paul Jones has written is enough to inspire you to not go it alone. Finding others in your community who share your mud-and-obstacle passion will bring you massive amounts of rewards and friendships that you could never achieve by yourself.

This begs the question: How do I find a group? In Appendix A, you'll find contact information for several large OCR groups. If none of those are close to you, you can do Facebook and Internet searches to see if one exists near you. If not, you may just have to be the one who makes it happen. Here are my best tips to do that.

CREATE A FACEBOOK GROUP. My suggestion is to create a Facebook group that is easy to find by name. Example: If you call the group "Tennessee Obstacle Racers," then people searching for an obstacle group in Tennessee will be more likely to find you than if you call your-selves "Mud Lovers of the South."

LIST A BASIC DESCRIPTION AND POST A FEW PHOTOS. This will be enough to show someone who comes across the page that you are legitimate. People will start to find you. You should make it a "closed" group, which means members have to be approved before they can join. Otherwise, you will get fake accounts and lots of spam. Don't make your group a "secret" Facebook group, though, because that means your group won't come up in a search.

INVITE PEOPLE TO JOIN. Whenever you are at a race, you will invariably make friends on the course or while enjoying a post-race beverage. Now, all you have to do is ask them, "Do you do these all the time?" Then add, "We have a Facebook group that I think you should join." Most people's reaction will be, "Great, I was looking for more people to do this with," or "We already have a small group that does these all the time. We'd love to hook up with more people."

▶ *Leaving the start line, you may be more confident if you have friends racing with you.*

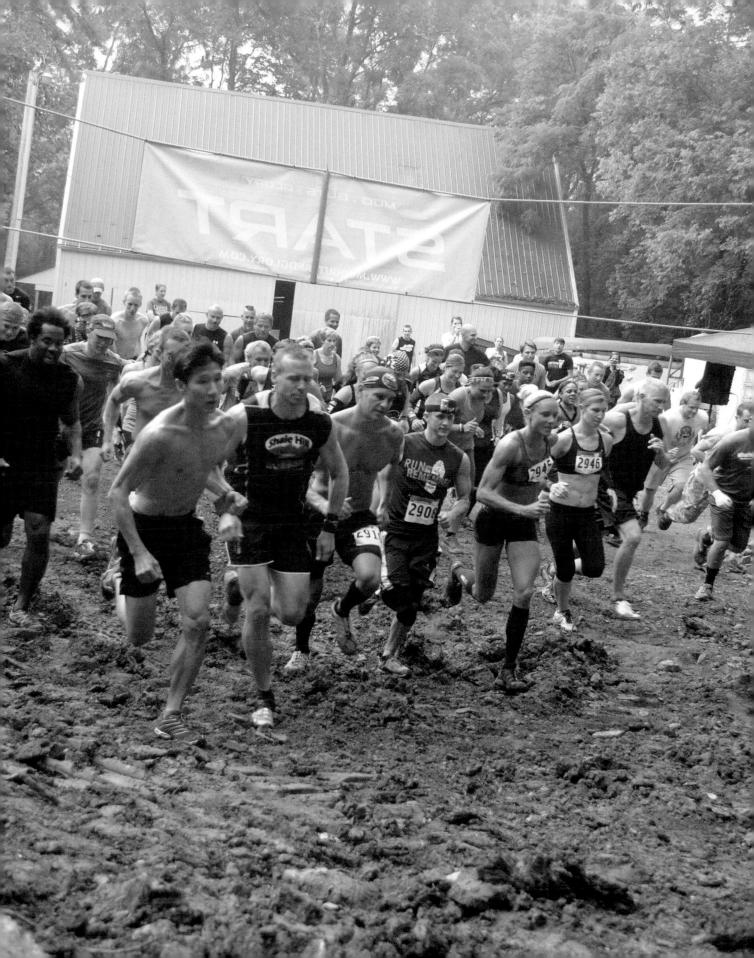

ENLIST HELP. Once you've made a few friends, give them access to the page as administrators so that you're not doing all the workload yourself. They will start to add people, and those people will start to add people, and before you know it, you will have one hundred members.

SHARE INFORMATION. One of the best things about a group like this is that you can create a race document. At the top of the group page, there is a link called "Files." Inside of that, there is a button that says "Create doc." You can then create a document that lists all the races coming up in your area. Everyone in the group has access and can add their names to races they plan on attending, or they can add new races as they find them.

When there's a race coming up, people can quickly view the race document and find people to carpool with to the race or just meet up with. It is also a great place to leave discount codes for other members.

There may already be a thriving group near you, but if not, now you have the tools to start one!

DOWN AND DIRTY TAKEAWAYS

- **Research.** Search Facebook for groups that already exist. There may be hundreds or thousands of people just like you waiting for you to join the fun.
- **Choose and use a name and logo.** Nothing attracts a crowd like a crowd. When people see your group name and logo on shirts, flags, and tents, they will come out of the woodwork.
- **Delegate.** You can't do it yourself. Many in the community will offer to help. Let them help with blog contributions, ideas, organizing training meet-ups, and everything else that the group wants to do.

Paul Jones found obstacle racing in its infancy, running his first race in 2010 and immediately getting hooked and helping to build the New England Spahtens from a small group of fans into the huge OCR community it is today. He now gets to work with both race directors and runners to help improve the OCR scene in New England for everyone. Jones and his merry brand of pranksters are constantly updating www.newenglandspahtens.com with blogs, race reviews, and other fun stuff.

▶ *The Corn Fed Spartans exemplified what it means to be a team as they carried this log through an entire course to honor a fallen comrade.*

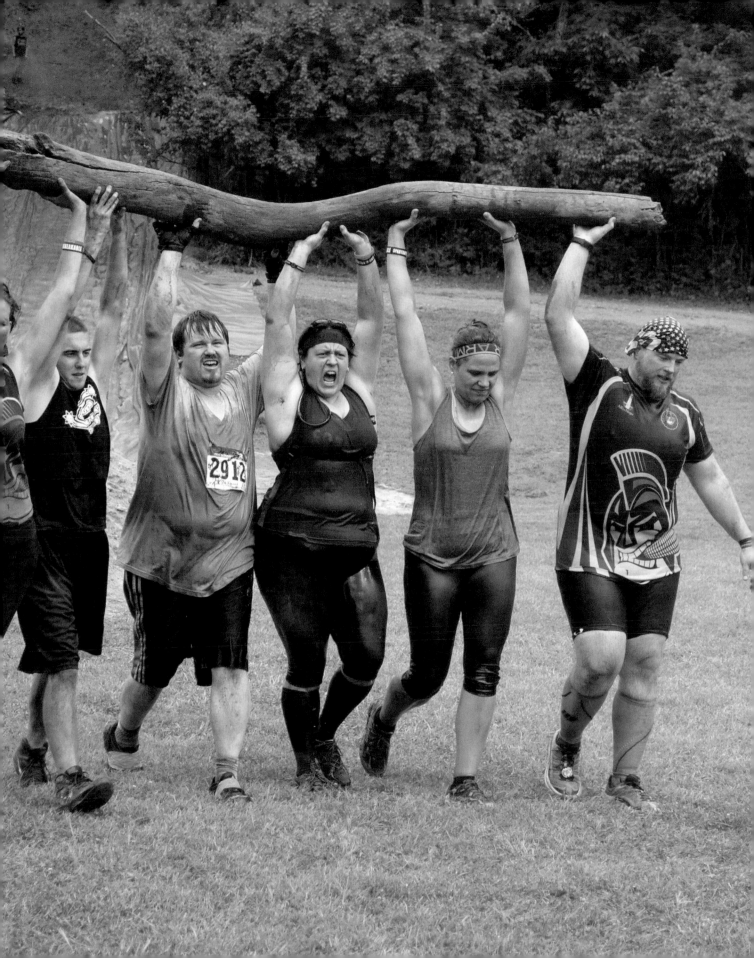

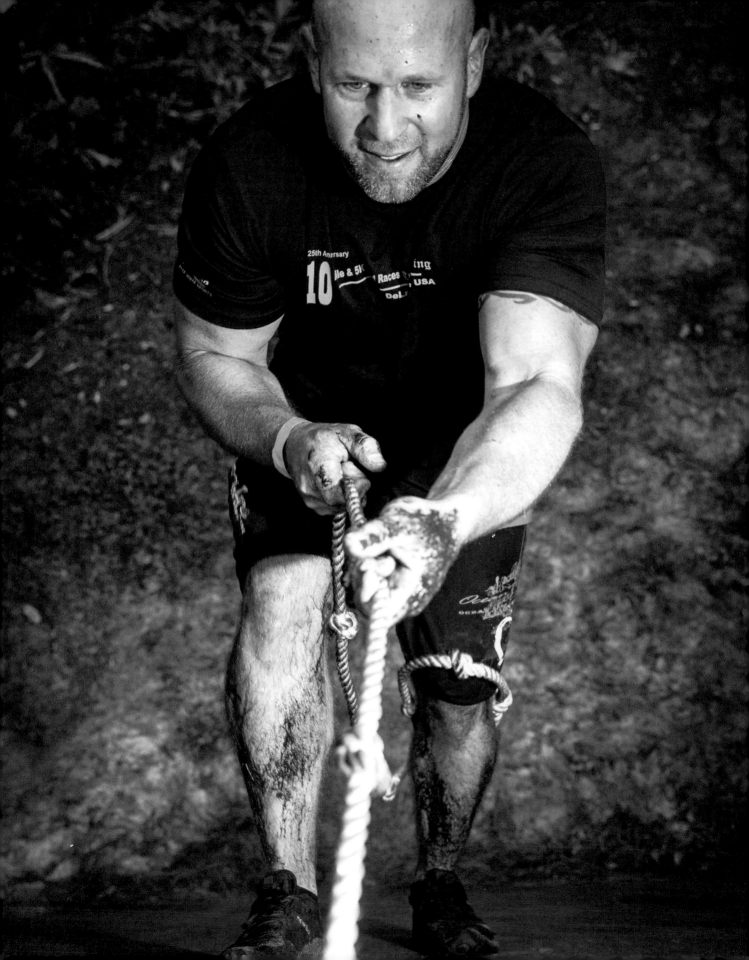

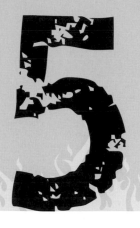

5 CHOOSING YOUR FIRST RACE AND REGISTERING

Commitment is doing the thing you said you were going to do, long after that feeling you had when you said you would do it has left you.

In the excitement of talking to friends and reading this book, you probably have committed in your mind to do your first race. It would be far too easy to let that feeling leave you and never actually sign up. The easiest way to keep that commitment is by "putting your money where your mouth is." Once that credit card has been charged, and you get that first confirmation email, you'll be fully committed to going. Sure, you could still back out on race day, but registering makes it so much easier to say to yourself, "I already paid for this thing. I may as well train and do it."

Choosing Your First Race

After reading the previous chapters and/or hearing stories about races being a disappointment or cancelling, you may have some additional doubts that don't have anything to do with your own abilities. I want to make it as easy as possible for you to choose your first race.

Let's start with the Big 3. They're the most likely to be coming to your area soon, and they give you the best chance to experience a high-quality event from top to bottom.

THE WARRIOR DASH

The Warrior Dash (WD) really lives up to its name. It is merely a dash of 3 miles (4.8 km) or less, with little to no terrain changes, and relatively simple obstacles. Anyone of any fitness level, including

◀ *Obstacles will test your mental and physical toughness.*

someone who hasn't gotten off the couch in a long time, could complete this event. It isn't designed to test you physically; it's designed to be a great time outside with your friends.

The only difference between someone very fit doing the WD and someone not so fit is time. A very fit person can do a WD in somewhere between 28 and 35 minutes. A person who runs and works out a couple times a week could do a WD in about 45 minutes. If you exercise less than that, it will just take you a little longer. You will still enjoy yourself throughout the course, and you and your friends will still enjoy a beverage, giant turkey leg, and great music afterward. The Warrior Dash is truly an entry-level event. Some people have even called it the "gateway drug" of OCR because it's most often the first experience that sucks them in and makes them want more. You can go to www.warriordash.com for more details and their complete schedule.

TOUGH MUDDER

A Tough Mudder (TM) is a very different event from the Warrior Dash, and it should be taken more seriously. For starters, Tough Mudders are 10 to 12 miles (16.1 to 19.3 km) long. For some racers, the hardest part of the race is just covering that distance. You can walk a majority of this if you like, but I would recommend that you're able to run at least 5 miles (8.1 km) with little trouble to get the maximum benefit. The obstacles in a TM will also be more challenging than those in a Warrior Dash.

Some of the obstacles in a TM are more mentally challenging. Jumping off a 12-foot (3.7 m) platform into a lake isn't hard physically, per se. However, if you're afraid of heights, it can be terrifying. Similarly is crawling through black drainage pipes. You're simply crawling on your hands and knees, which almost anyone can do. But to some people, not seeing light on the other side is a huge barrier for them to get through.

I'll take a moment here to mention electric shock obstacles. These are the ones that seem to frighten people the most because of the fear of the unknown. Here's what I can tell you, having done at least six obstacle races that have had electric shocks. Sometimes you feel nothing, sometimes it's a little sting, and other times it's a big sting, which can in fact knock you unconscious for a moment. I have had all of those experiences, and I didn't die. At the end of the day, electric obstacles are more of a mental challenge than a physical one for most people. That said, speak with a medical professional first, especially if you have any heart issues.

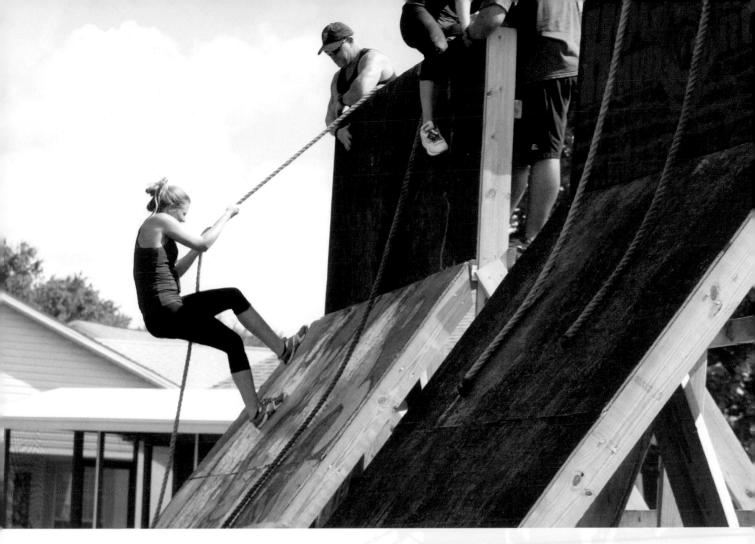

▲ *Sometimes the walls will have ropes to help; other times they won't.*

One of the biggest themes in a TM is teamwork. In the pledge at the start of the race, you and your fellow Mudders will recite, "I put teamwork and camaraderie before my course time." This is the biggest reason why I believe even a first-timer can complete a TM. Friends, and quite often, complete strangers, will assist you in completing the obstacles. They'll put a knee or back out for you to stand on, hold down a cargo net for you to climb over, and hold barbed wire up for you to crawl under.

"I put teamwork and camaraderie before my course time."

The more challenging obstacles at TM, which you are on your own for, are things such as hanging rings, called "Hangin' Tough," or the inverted monkey bars, which they call "Funky Monkey." As a newbie, you may not be able to complete these obstacles. (I personally have gotten farther each time I have tried, but I have yet to complete either one myself.) There's

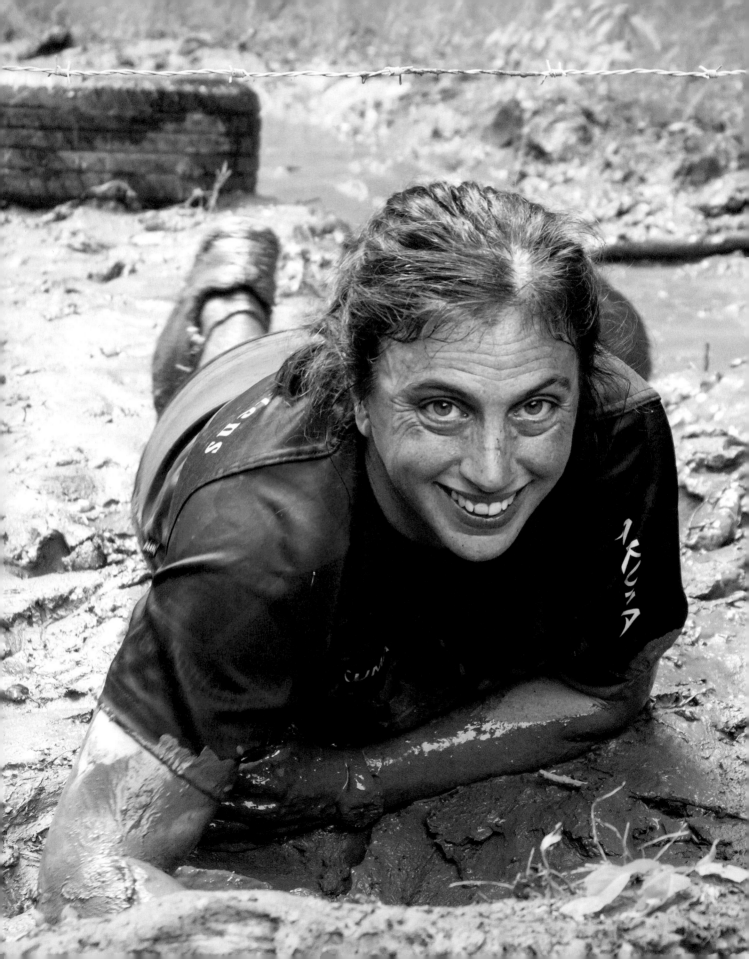

no penalty for not completing them. For the two I just mentioned, you simply fall into the water and continue on with your race. Now, if it's really cold out, it's an additional burden to be wet and cold. But at least you won't have to do burpees or some other punishment for not completing the obstacle.

A fit athlete will likely complete a TM in 2 to 3 hours. The average person will complete one in 3 to 5 hours. Other people will take considerably longer. If you're not concerned about setting speed records at your first TM, I would say put on a backpack, fill it with food and nutrition gels, and have a go at it. TMs have plenty of water stations to keep you hydrated, but they may not have bananas or other food at every stop.

I believe that you can train for three to four months and have Tough Mudder be your virgin mission into OCR land, but if you have a Warrior Dash or something easier coming into town sooner than the TM, go ahead and get your feet wet that way. Go to www.toughmudder.com for more information and schedules.

SPARTAN RACE

Spartan Race has three core types of distances in their race series: the Sprint, the Super, and the Beast. If you want a fun day in the mud, do *not* sign up for a Super or Beast as your first mud run/obstacle course race.

Having said that, their entry-level race, a Spartan Sprint, is an awesome way to introduce yourself to the world of obstacle course racing. You'll be challenged, you'll have fun, and you can push yourself in a big way. This may not make sense at first, but a 5- to 7-mile (8.1 to 11.3 km) Spartan Sprint can be as physically challenging as a 10-mile (16.1 km) Tough Mudder. You'll also experience as much camaraderie as you will in a TM. At a Spartan Race, the runners next to you are just as likely to help you over a wall, through an obstacle, or share their last Power Bar with you even though they are wearing timing chips on their sneakers.

Typically, Spartan Sprints' obstacles require you to carry heavy things, which work your upper body harder than Warrior Dashes or even Tough Mudders. There are typically sandbag carries, bucket carries, or large cement stone carries. I have seen people of all fitness levels

◄ *It always helps to smile.*

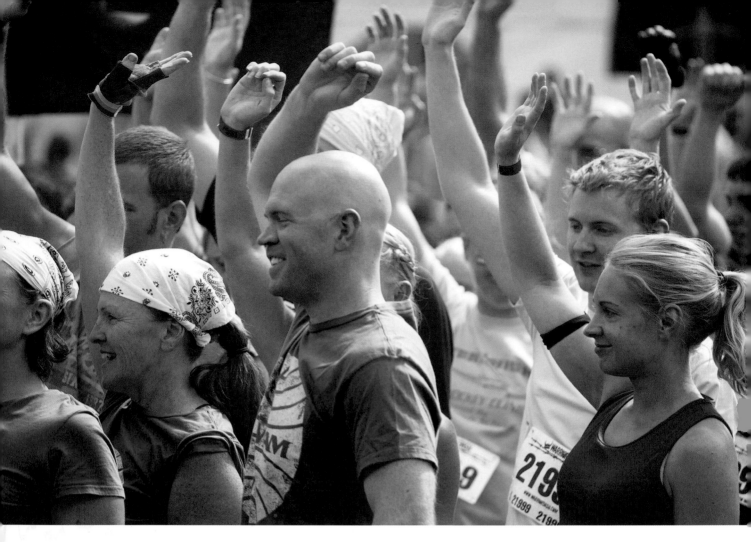

▲ *Raise your hand if you are ready to race.*

complete these obstacles, though. You may have to stop and rest several times during one of these "carries," but you can still get it done.

Elite athletes typically finish a Spartan Sprint in 38 to 45 minutes. The average person will take somewhere between 1:15 and 2 hours. Because Spartan Race distances and terrain vary greatly, your times may or may not fall within those ranges, whether it is your first race or your tenth.

The Spartan Race's second type of race, the Super Races, are advertised as 8-plus miles (12.9-plus km), and the Beasts are advertised as 12-plus miles (19.3-plus km). I qualified that by "advertised as" because Spartan has been known to play with these mileages and make the races longer.

They've also been known to make the terrain more difficult than any other race series. For example, at the 2013 Virginia Super Spartan, the elite winners took longer to complete the course than they had any other previous Spartan Beast race! The Spartan Races also have the most challenging obstacles of any race series, plus they enforce burpee penalties if a racer misses an obstacle, which sap tons of energy and confidence. The Spartan Race is easily the most challenging of the Big 3.

At the end of the day, your experience will be what you put into it. Some people have done a Big 3 race as their first race and stated it was the greatest time in their lives. Other people who show up with certain expectations will want their money back.

NON-BIG 3 RACES

Next, I want to talk about selecting a race other than the Big 3 for your first event, or how to select your second and third

event after you have done one or all of the Big 3 and want to try more.

In recent years, more than 250 different race series have popped up in the United States. In the U.K., there are 80 race organizations putting on 170 events. In Australia, there are 40 race companies with 60–65 races per year. How do you know if you're going to get a great race with fun obstacles, or if you are going to be sorely disappointed? Here are some important points to watch out for.

LOOK CLOSELY AT THE RACE ORGANIZER'S WEBSITE. What, they have no website? Experience tells us that a Facebook launch before a website is live spell trouble. Also, what do the photos and videos on their website and social media look like? Are the photos advertising the race actually old race photos from another race? Is their video stolen material? As a new race director, it's tough to show your stuff before your first event, but you can do it without ripping off other race series.

CHECK OUT THEIR EVENT CALENDAR. Are they promising many events, all over the country? Rather than being a sign of encouragement that they are doing well, this should be an immediate red flag—especially if they haven't already hosted their first event! An additional red flag is listing race cities and dates with no locations. Time and time again, I've seen these dates eventually disappear off their websites when they don't get enough people registered. Have they posted both Saturday *and* Sunday race days? This is another red flag. These companies expect to sell enough tickets to host two days of racing, when even the Big 3 don't do multiday events in some cities. A new race that does it right starts out small. They don't make unrealistic promises. They produce local events, and after garnering success, they start to slowly grow and add additional dates within their state or region of the country.

ASK QUESTIONS. Post a question on a race organizer's Facebook page or email them directly. Do they get back to you in a timely manner? Does the response look professional, or does it look like it was typed with the syntax of a teenager texting? If something seems fishy or unprofessional, it usually is.

CONSULT A GROUP. In chapter 4, I talked about finding or starting an OCR group. These groups are going to be your best bet for immediate knowledge and feedback. The members of these groups will have great insight on races—either because they have already run that particular race, or because they know and are already working with that race director directly to help put on a top-quality event.

CHECK OCR WEBSITES. The websites in Appendix B on page 217 will have tons of reviews available.

USE GOOGLE. When all else fails, Google is your friend. Simply typing in "<race name> review" will help you immensely.

Let me be clear, I'm not saying "Never sign up for brand-new races." Plenty of new races do an adequate job the first time around, have some bumps in the road early on, listen to feedback, and continue to improve and become thriving series in OCR. However, they aren't the ones boasting to be the "toughest day of your life" and posting nationwide dates, thinking they're the next big thing.

If you don't mind gambling a few hours of your time, a race is nearby, the cost of entry is manageable or discounted, and you set your expectations low, you really can't lose. It's when you pay a pretty penny, drive several hours, and have

▶ *You may not look at tires the same way again after an obstacle race.*

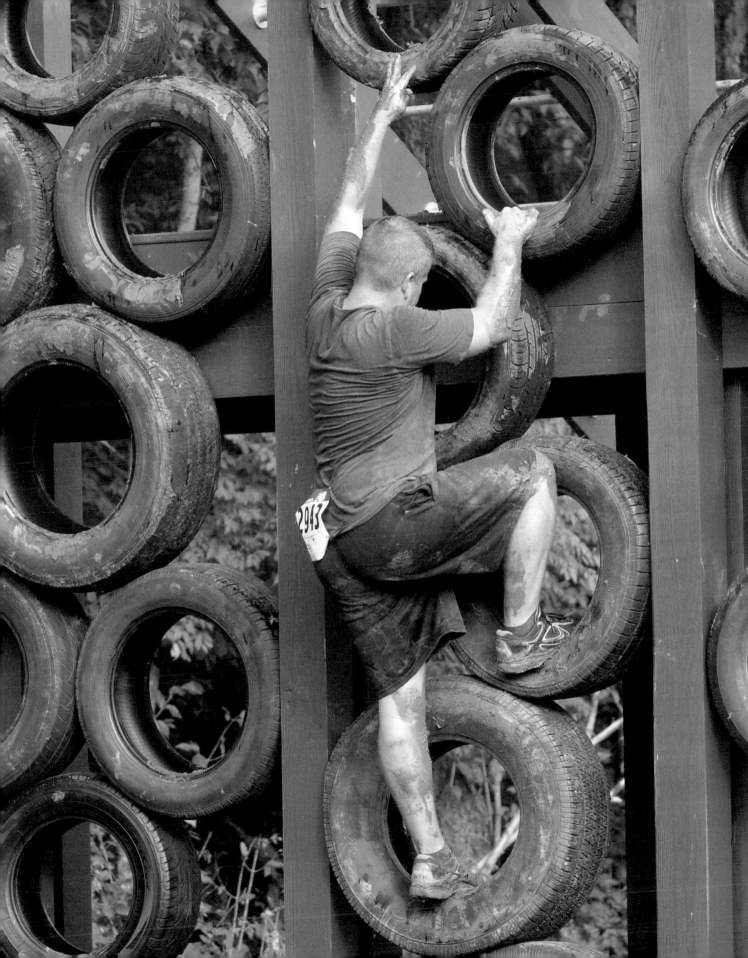

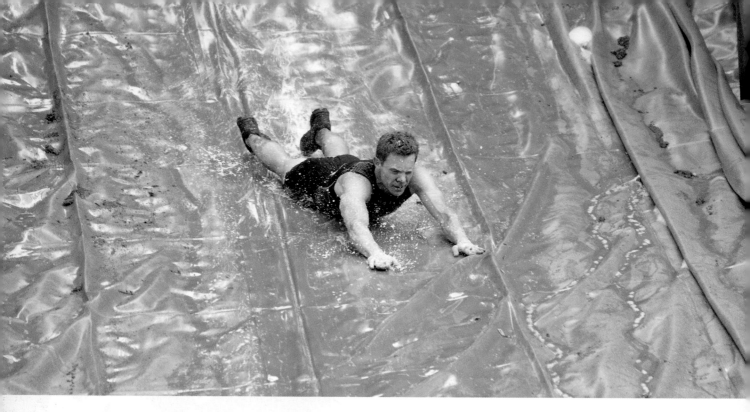

▲ *Some consider Slip and Slides more fun than obstacles.*

to pay accommodation costs that you'll be kicking yourself if the race is bad or cancels with no refunds.

Note: Some portions of text from this chapter were taken from http://obstacle racingmedia.com/editorial/which-new-races-should-i-avoid written by Matt B. Davis and Paul Jones, which was first published August 16, 2013.

DOWN AND DIRTY TAKEAWAYS

The Warrior Dash, sometimes called the "OCR gateway drug," is an excellent choice for most people attempting their first obstacle course race. It's a great way to get your feet wet.

- **Ask questions.** Post questions to race organizers about newer races that you are unsure about. Their timeliness and professionalism (or lack thereof) will tell you whether their race is worth registration for.
- **Start today.** Don't wait until you are "ready" or "in shape" to register. Pick a race, mark your calendar, and give yourself a goal to shoot for by registering.

▶ *How would you attack this one?*

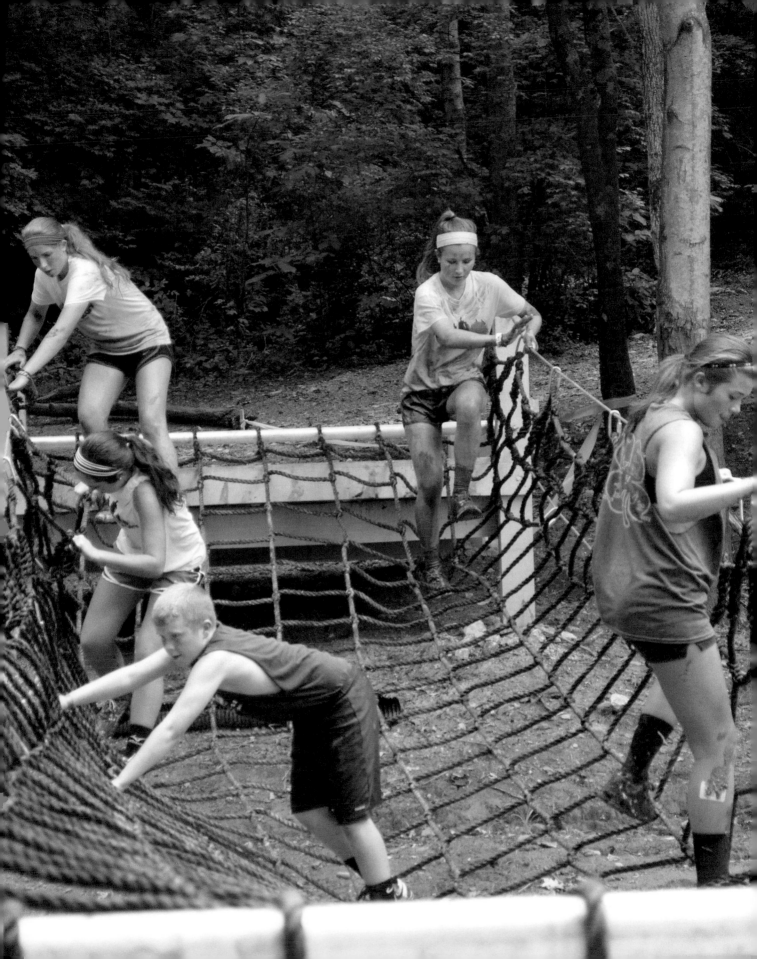

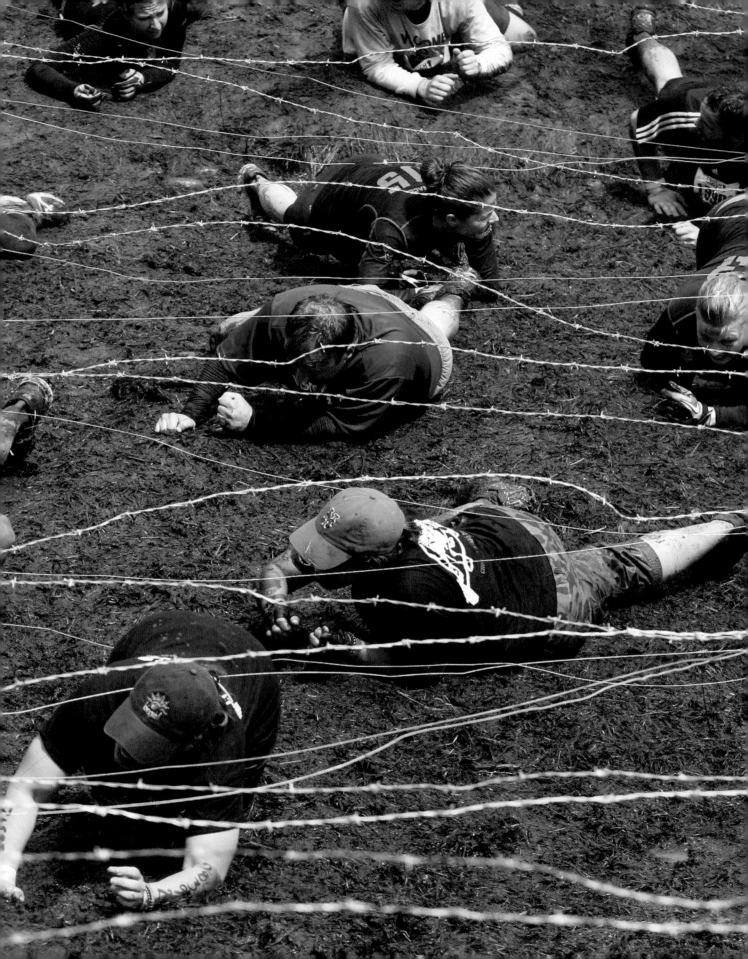

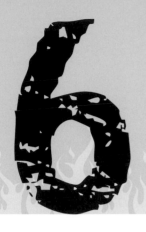

OTHER KEY POINTS FOR NEWCOMERS

Included in this chapter are some key points to registering for and preparing to participate in obstacle course races that are not mentioned in other parts of this book. They are invaluable pieces of wisdom gained from experience from countless obstacle course races and obstacle course racers. These important notes will help you immensely in your obstacle course racing journey.

Time of Day

When you race can have a huge impact on the kind of experience you have. At almost every race series, the first heat of the day is reserved for the "elites." If you aren't an elite, and if you're concerned at all with how long the course will take you, you're going to want to run at the next possible heat or the one immediately after that. For a safe bet, choose the 9 a.m. race time.

If you race in the middle of the day, or sometimes even as early as 10 a.m., there's a good chance that you'll experience backups at one or more obstacles from all the people on the course. Some people view these backups as a chance to rest from the running and to chit-chat with their friends. This will drive other people crazy, and they might even want to just skip that obstacle.

Another advantage to racing early is that this will often make for an easier course. Racing in the morning means thousands of racers haven't yet muddied up slippery obstacles or made mud pits even harder to get across. In later races, the course will certainly be at its muddiest.

◄ *Be prepared to get dirty.*

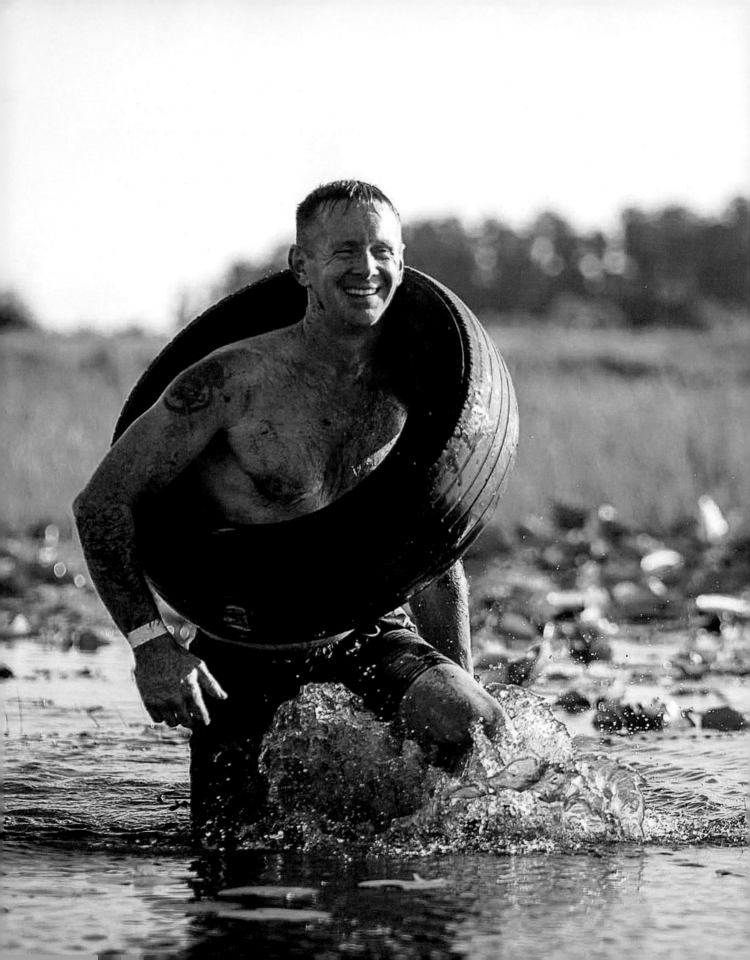

The early waves typically sell out the fastest, so you may have no choice but to race in a later wave. If that happens to you, you can console yourself with the thought that often the last waves of the day are actually less crowded than the morning or afternoon, because almost everyone is done. So you may not experience lines at the obstacles.

Many races do not strictly enforce the time you race, so you can often "sneak in" to an earlier (or later) wave. But I can't personally guarantee that will work.

Volunteering

Did you know that you might be able to race for free by assisting for a few hours race day morning? Most races employ this policy as a way to get additional help. Most of the time, by showing up at 6 a.m. and helping until noon, you can run in an afternoon wave that very same day for free.

Some races even pay for help. For example, a large race series such as Spartan will pay a small stipend for working in certain shifts and give you a free race. If you don't mind getting up really early, this is an awesome way to save some money and become really involved.

Beyond getting a free race, service can be its own reward. Greeting participants in the morning at registration with a smile, cheering them on at obstacles, or putting medals around hundreds if not thousands of necks can provide an experience that you'll never forget.

Volunteering can also have some very happy unexpected consequences. I know people who have made lifelong friends, found their life mates, or gotten job offers as a result of being OCR volunteers.

Most race websites will have a direct link for volunteering. Many times it can be found on their FAQ page or as a part of your race registration. If you cannot find the info you are looking for, simply contact the race directly, and they will be happy to tell you how you can help.

Hazards

I'll start with the worst. There have been a few catastrophic events at obstacle races. A few people have died, and others have had life-changing injuries. When you look at the millions of people who have participated to date in the United States, the number of catastrophic events is tiny, at around 0.0003 percent. There have been a few major neck injuries due

◄ *Opt for synthetic materials when choosing race clothing. Never wear cotton; it is very unpleasant to wear when wet.*

to falls, and the deaths that I'm aware of as of this writing were from heatstroke or drowning. Every race company will tell you they put safety first. The majority of them do a great job. When done right, you'll find helpful volunteers at every obstacle. At water obstacles, they'll have certified lifeguards, EMTs, and other safety personnel in the water and on land ready to help at a moment's notice.

Being overly cautious is never a bad thing. If you're at a race, and you see a wall or other wooden obstacle that looks unstable, don't get on it. If you see water obstacles and not enough safety personnel, don't do that obstacle, and don't get in the water. Also, bring it to someone's attention as soon as possible because you may be able to help the next participant. Sometimes, a person is too tired or too caught up in the moment to be as aware as they should be of their surroundings.

What to Wear and Bring

The questions of what to bring and what to wear are probably the most asked by newbies.

Opinions vary widely on what *brands* to wear or what *kinds* of nutrition to bring. But I can tell you about 95 percent of the experienced OCR veterans I know will agree on the following things.

- **DON'T WEAR COTTON.** None, not a stitch of it, not even underwear. One thing is sure, no matter the race, you *will* be wet and muddy. Cotton becomes extremely heavy—a lot heavier than you think—so you don't want any of it on your person. You may not own a lot of synthetic "racing clothing." (I didn't when I started.) Luckily, many stores sell this stuff fairly cheaply. My first few races were in cold weather, so I had to borrow compression tights and a long-sleeved shirt from a friend. Slowly, but surely, I bought more and more clothing, and now I'm prepared for any season.

- **MORE LAYERS DON'T MEAN MORE WARMTH.** Because you're going to be wet and muddy, layering up will not help, and it will in fact weigh you down. In colder weather, I suggest wearing two layers at max on any part of your body.

- **LESS CAN BE MORE.** Some athletes are brave enough to wear next to nothing on race day. Men choose to wear shorts only, and women will wear

▶ *You won't always get this wet, but you will get wet.*

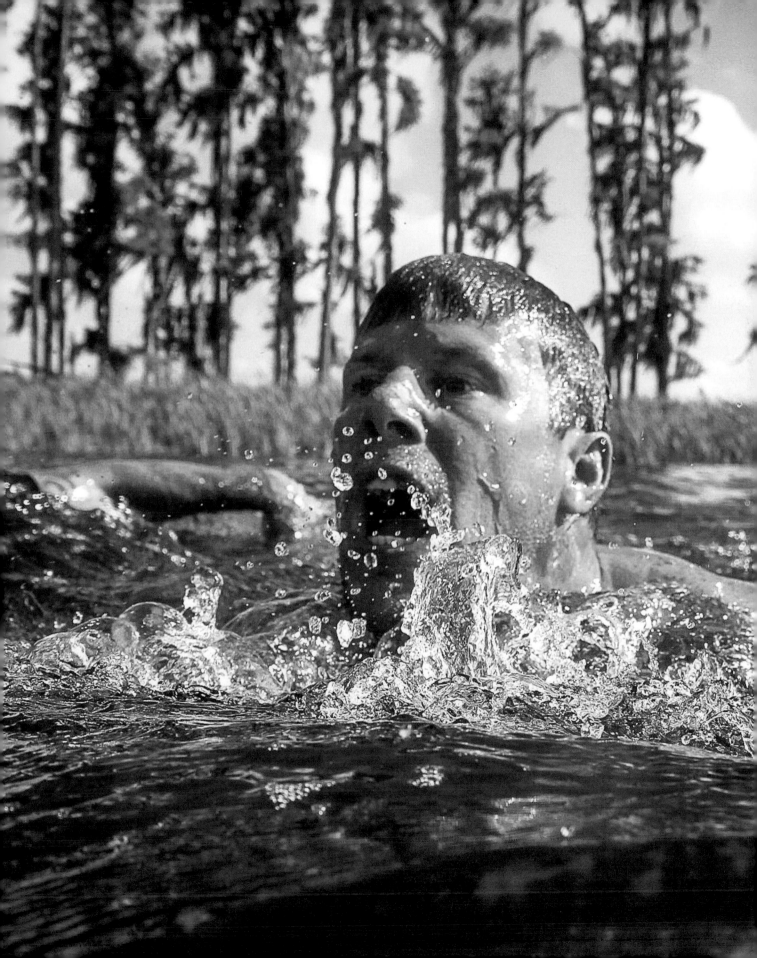

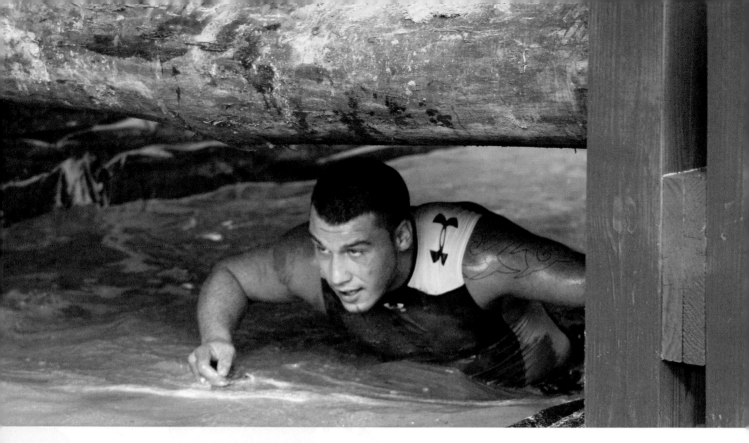

▲ *When it comes to clothing, less is more.*

shorts and a sports bra only—even on the coldest of days. The theory is that skin dries faster than clothing will, and the body will heat itself faster.

A trick I found that can work is a "best of both worlds" situation. If it's an especially cold day, I remove my outer layer (or only layer) before submerging myself in a water obstacle. Then I can put the dry layer back on after getting out of the water.

Let's look at Tough Mudder's Arctic Enema (ice bath) obstacle as an example. If it's a frigid morning, I'll most likely leave the start line with two layers on my upper body, wearing a long-sleeved compression shirt over a synthetic tank top. Approaching this obstacle, I set one or both of my shirts down on the ground, jump into the ice water, and then run back to put on my dry layers of clothing. Often, a volunteer or spectator will even hold your clothing if you ask nicely.

- **CONSIDER GLOVES.** The only time I recommend gloves is if the temperature is 35° F (2° C) or below on race day. This is 100 percent for warmth purposes and not because it will make obstacles easier. Implementing the previously mentioned, "best of both worlds" situation, I take the gloves off when approaching water or mud, and then put them back on to keep my hands warm while running to the next obstacle.

- **CHOOSE THE RIGHT SHOES.** Most race directors will recommend that you wear a pair of shoes that you do not care about, and then donate them at the end. That would be great if you only plan on running one race. If you plan on doing this more than once, it can be very expensive. There are no less than 1 zillion blogs (I counted) on who makes the best shoes for OCR. As of this writing, a few companies are actually releasing "obstacle course racing shoes." The verdict is not out yet on whether they will be any good. For now, I say run in whatever sneakers you have. If you have trail shoes of any kind, they would be preferred over a straight street shoe, but a street shoe will work fine, too, for your first race. As you do this more, talk to other racers, and try different things, and you'll find what works best for you.

- **BRING NUTRITION.** If the race is 5k or shorter, such as a Warrior Dash, you most likely won't need nutrition. Remember, you'll only be out there for a short amount of time—around an hour, and that time won't require a snack. If the race is longer, it can never hurt to bring a little nutrition—*even if the race advertises there will be some food at the water stations*. It's better to have it and not need it than the other way around. Sometimes the race does not supply it at every station, they forget to get it out there until later in the day, or they run out. You can wear a SPIbelt (or other similar brands), which is a small personal item belt that allows you to carry small items and will fit several bars, GUs, or gels. Another way racers have solved the nutrition problem is to simply duct tape items onto their person.

- **DON'T CARRY WATER.** I don't recommend carrying water for any race unless the race is more than 10 miles (16.1 km)—such as the Iron Warrior Dash, Spartan Ultra Beast, or certain Spartan Supers—or if you expect you will be on the course for more than 2 hours. This doesn't include Tough Mudder races, which typically provide water every 1 to 3 miles (1.6 to 4.8 km). If you plan on taking your time and making a day of it, feel free to wear a CamelBak water bottle. Just know that you may have a harder time getting

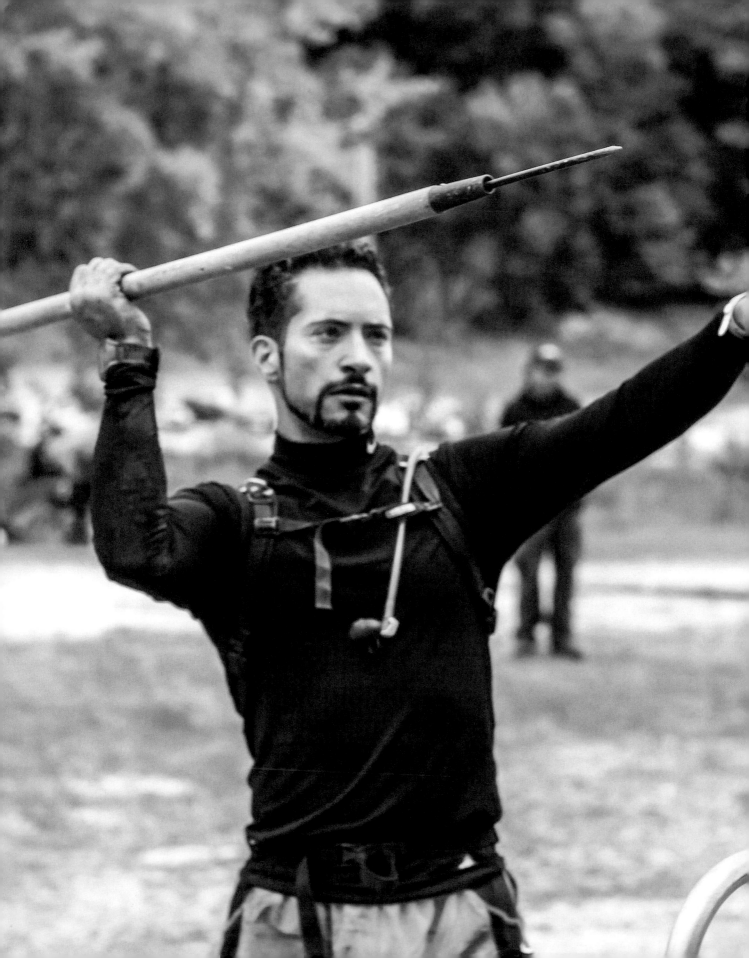

under barbed wire with your backpack on. Or plan on ditching your water source to the side before a barbed wire crawl then walking back to get it after you complete the obstacle.

Before you go to a race, read the racer/athlete information emails carefully. The race companies will typically give you lots of information on the kinds of aid they are providing and what they recommend you bring.

- **BRING CASH; IT'S KING.** Often these races take place in remote areas. There is no ATM on site, and you may need cash for parking, food, beverages, and/or bag check.

- **PACK DRY CLOTHES AND A TOWEL.** When you're done with the race, whether you want to spend some time enjoying the spoils of your accomplishments with your friends or you want to just jump in your car and leave, you'll want some dry clothes. Be sure to pack dry clothes to change into, including a fresh pair of socks and shoes. You'll also want to bring a towel to clean off and dry off with and a garbage bag to throw the muddy clothes into so you don't dirty up your

DOWN AND DIRTY TAKEAWAYS

- **Run early.** The early bird gets the worm. Run in the morning if you want to avoid lines and backups at obstacles. The middle of the day typically has the most crowded waves.

- **Race for free.** Check each OCR's website to find out how volunteering can earn you a chance to race with no money down.

- **Don't wear cotton.** Wear anything but cotton if you want to have a pleasant race experience.

vehicle on the way home. The "shower" facilities at races can vary widely. Some have awesome high- powered water areas, while others have lame setups, which offer little more than a trickle. Experienced racers know to find the nearest body of water to jump into after the race.

◄ *Ready, steady, aim, fire!*

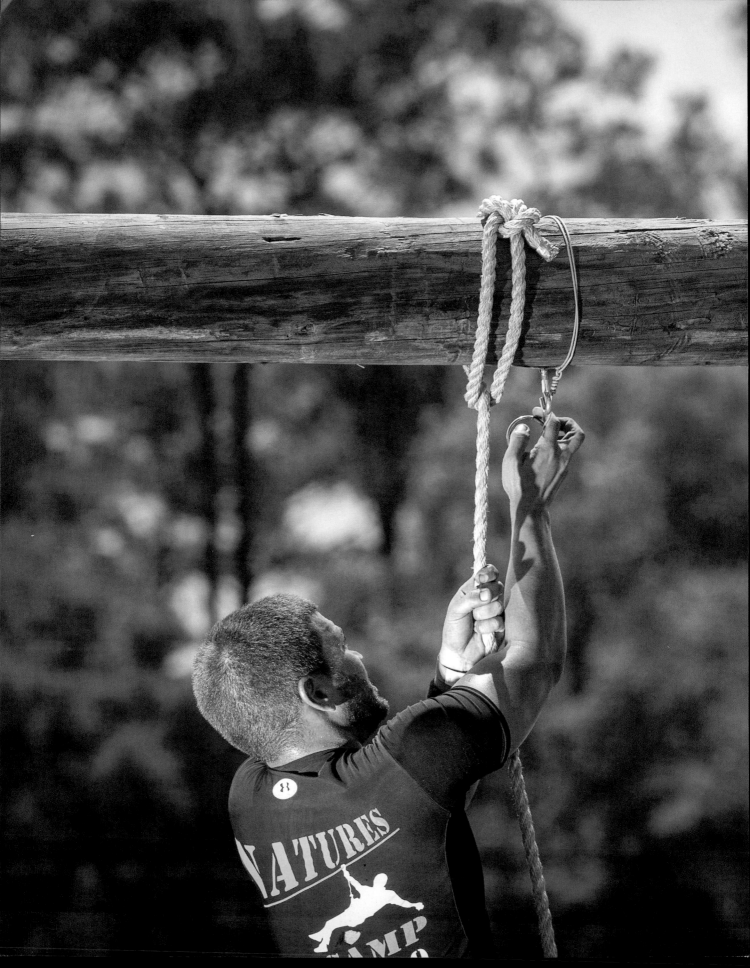

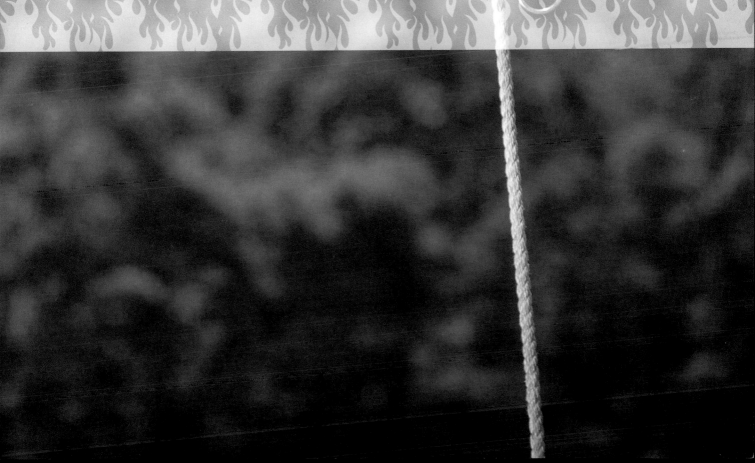

PART II

TRAINING FOR PERFORMANCE AND CONQUERING THE OBSTACLES

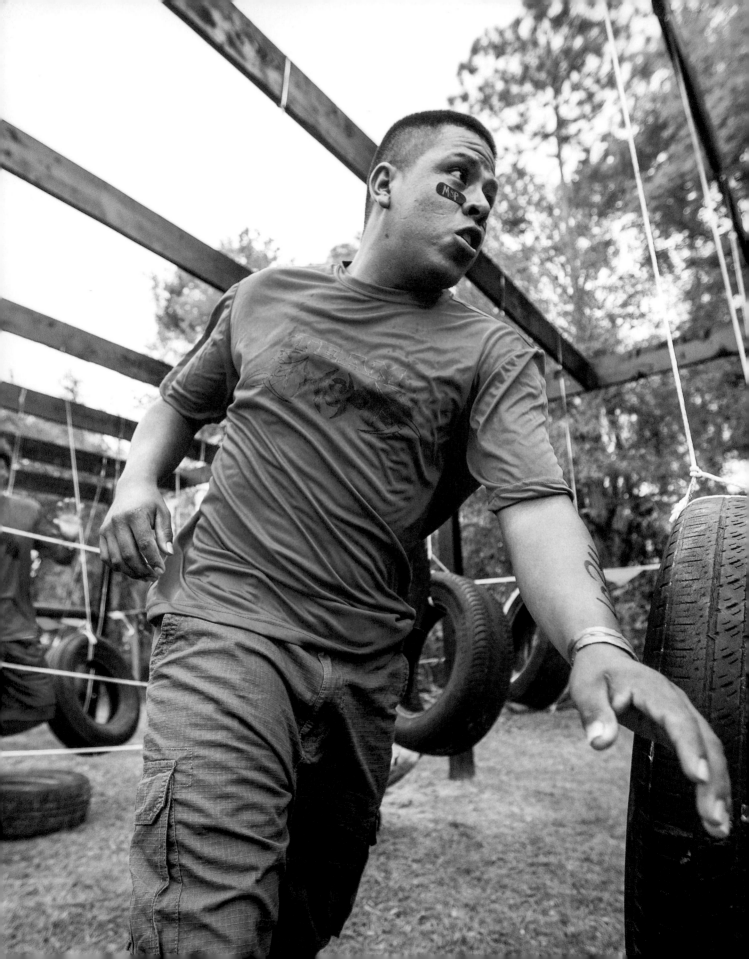

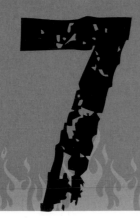

7 GET OFF THE COUCH AND RUN YOUR FIRST MILE

You'll encounter a variety of obstacles during your race, but training begins the same way for everyone: getting off the couch and starting to run.

In fall 2011, I was a thirty-nine-year-old man who was not physically active. Sure, I played flag football, which required some physical exertion, and I played organized softball, which required even less. But I hadn't lifted a weight or been to the gym since I was a teenager. I hadn't run more than a mile since 1985.

No one would have called me obese; I was average. As a mesomorph, I never had huge fluctuations in weight; I just sort of maintained. Then I saw a video for a Tough Mudder race. It was *intense*, showing men and women running through fire, jumping into cold water, and crawling through mud. I watched a training video of a man who dumped cold water on himself then ran barefoot in the snow for a few miles.

All of this was pretty scary. I thought maybe, one day, a few years from now, I could do it. Then a few weeks later, a friend of mine and I were writing goals we wanted to accomplish in the next year. One of the things he wrote down was "complete a Tough Mudder." This friend is older than me and in worse shape. If he could do it, I certainly could. I registered online a few days later. The race was advertised as 10 to 12 miles (16.1 to 19.3 km), so I found a training program for a half marathon. I was under the impression that if you were going to train for a race that long, you had to run 10 to 12 miles (16.1 to 19.3 km) several times a week. I had barely run a mile, so it was rather daunting.

◄ *You'll encounter a variety of obstacles during your race, but training begins the same way for everyone: getting off the couch and starting to run.*

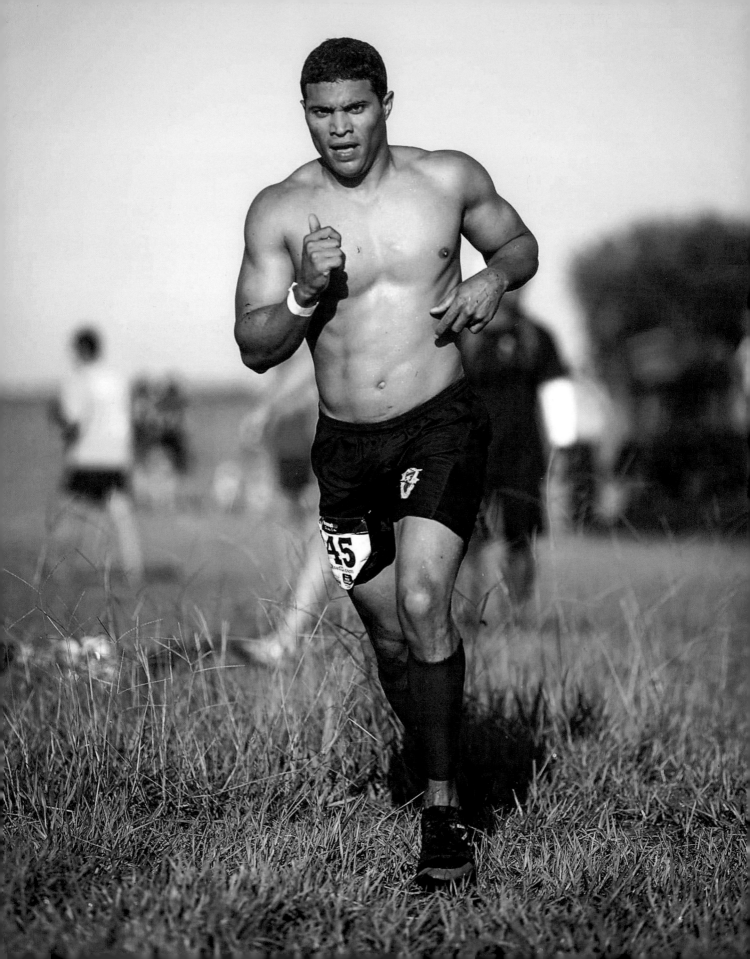

It turns out that you don't have to run anywhere near that much. You can start out at 1 to 2 miles (1.6 to 3.2 km) a day, and then as time goes on, you try 3 miles (4.8 km), then 4 (6.4 km). Slowly, you build your long runs. The first Saturday, you run 5 miles (8.1 km). The next Saturday, you run 6 miles (9.7 km). You want to consistently run 2 to 4 miles (3.2 to 6.4 km) a day a few times a week. It's slow and steady, and it will build your confidence.

When I began training, I thought 1 mile (1.6 km) was sufficient. Three laps around the park was a mile, so I got out there and started running. It took me somewhere close to 12 minutes, and it was painful.

The next day, I encountered my neighbor Chris walking his dog. He asked me what I was doing because he had never known me to be a runner. I told him that I was training for a Tough Mudder. He also decided to register for the race, and he joined me during my training regimen. This was key for my routine, because Chris became my running buddy as we prepared for the Tough Mudder.

We would text each other on running days to plan when we would meet up.

Having another person to hold me accountable made all the difference. There have been plenty of times during and since that I had planned to run by myself and found an excuse not to—too hot, too cold, want to be with family, don't feel like it, need a nap, etc. Having someone to meet with makes me accountable, and it also adds a social element and made my training more enjoyable. Of course, one can still find excuses not to train, but it's harder when you know someone is expecting you.

Chris and I began running 2 to 3 miles (3.2 to 4.8 km) a day. I could barely keep up with him because he would be going at a "conversational pace," and I was breathing heavily as we were talking and running. Then one day, it happened.

We went for our normal loop with two other neighborhood friends. When we got to the stopping point at the end of the loop, something took over. Something told me to keep going. I whizzed past my friends and said, "I'm going to keep going." I ran faster and farther than I had in years. I was smiling from ear to ear. I loved it. I thought, "I could keep going forever!"

I ran for a total of 4.5 miles (7.2 km) that day, a new personal record. I know

◄ *Get out and start running.*

I could have gone farther, but something told me to keep building my distance slowly, so I reined it in.

A few weeks into my running regimen, I spoke to a friend who was an avid runner. I called him for advice on purchasing new running shoes. He recommended a book called *Born to Run*. To say this book changed my life would not be an exaggeration. I ran almost every day, and before I went to bed at night, I would dig in to *Born to Run*. Everything in the book was fascinating: The author's journey, the characters he meets along the way, and the story of the Tarahumara Indians had me riveted. It also motivated me to get out there every day and run farther.

How should you tackle running that first mile? First, consider downloading an app for your smartphone that can keep track of your progress. There are many free applications, and I personally prefer the RunKeeper app. Along with the basic features of tracking your time, distance, and elevation, it can give you a training program for races. For example, there are built-in programs for your first 5k, your first half marathon, or a 4-hour marathon. RunKeeper also makes it easy to sync with a watch if you prefer to download to a computer later rather than your smartphone. Similar apps offer the same basic features, including MapMyRun and Daily Mile. Your preferences may vary.

If you don't like to run with your phone, you might instead consider a GPS watch. But my assumption is that as a beginner, you're more likely to already own a phone, and you don't want to wait to buy a GPS watch to get started.

The only way to get yourself out there to run is to do it. Pick a day, and make it happen. It could be today, tomorrow morning, or tomorrow after work.

I suggest not thinking about getting to 5k, 5 miles (8.1 km), or whatever the distance of your first race is going to be. Just choose to run today and go for it, regardless of the distance. If 1 mile (1.6 km) seems daunting, choose a shorter goal. Pick an easy goal, such as one lap around the block. Run at an easy pace. If you feel like you can go farther, run another lap. If you're spent after the one lap, stop and try again tomorrow. Keep trying until you can make that second lap. Then increase your distance. Keep challenging yourself to go farther.

I strongly encourage that you find a buddy to run with. You probably already

▶ *Be ready to get filthy.*

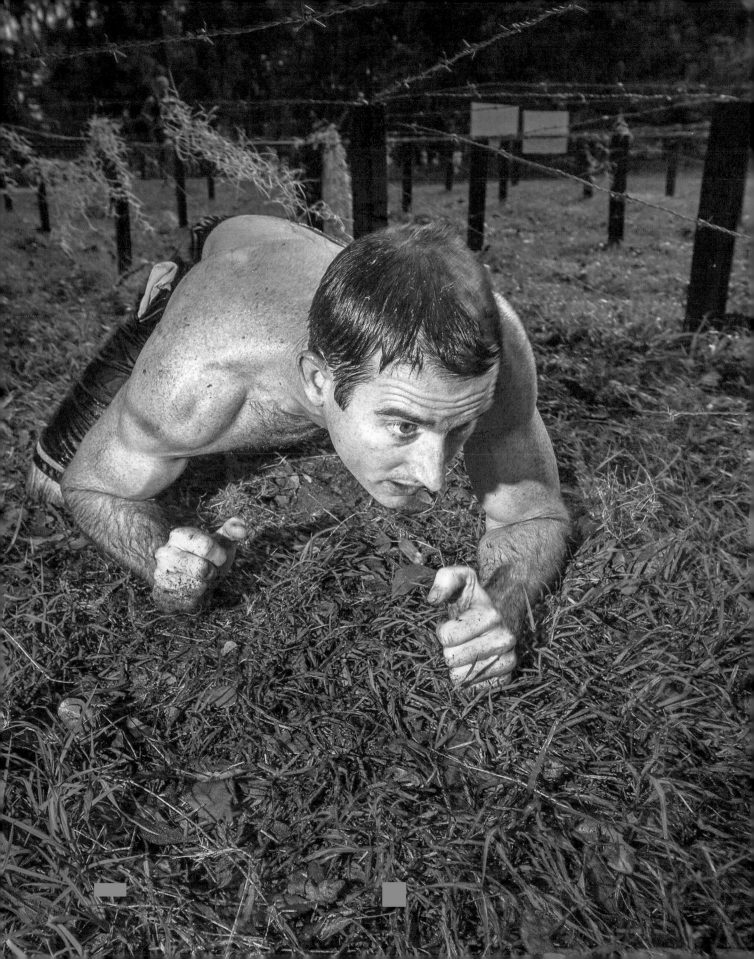

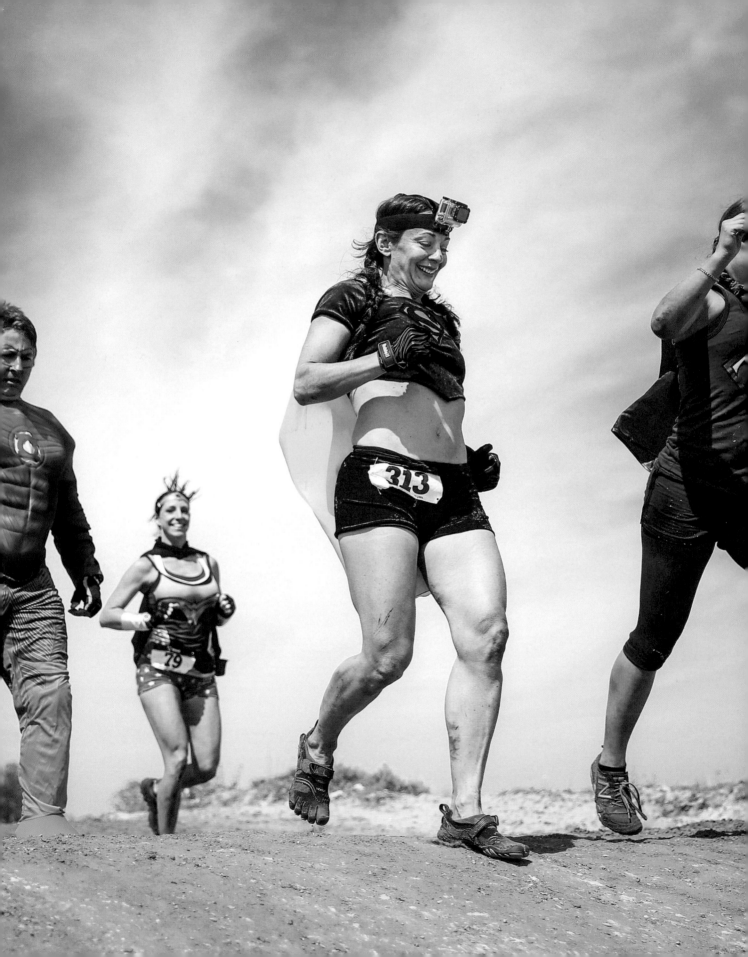

know someone who runs a lot. Ask him or her to go with you. Don't be afraid that you'll be "too slow for them." When I started, many times I went with a friend or a group of a few people. They were always happy to accommodate a slower pace. I am now willing to do the same when I run with beginners.

Speaking of groups, there is a great site called www.meetup.com. It is free to join. You can search for running groups in your area, and you'll likely find many running-focused groups nearby. Surely, a few of them will have meeting times that work for your schedule. Again, don't worry about being the slowest in the group. You won't be the only new person or the only one who may want a slower pace; everyone has his/her own individual goals.

DOWN AND DIRTY TAKEAWAYS

- **Get an app.** Download RunKeeper or a similar application on your phone to track your time, distance, and progress.
- **Start somewhere.** Choose to walk/run some distance. It can be one block or 1 mile (1.6 km). Pick one and go.
- **Find a friend.** A running buddy can make running more fun and also help hold you accountable.

◄ *Training with a friend is a great way to maintain motivation. You may find friends to join you on your first obstacle course race.*

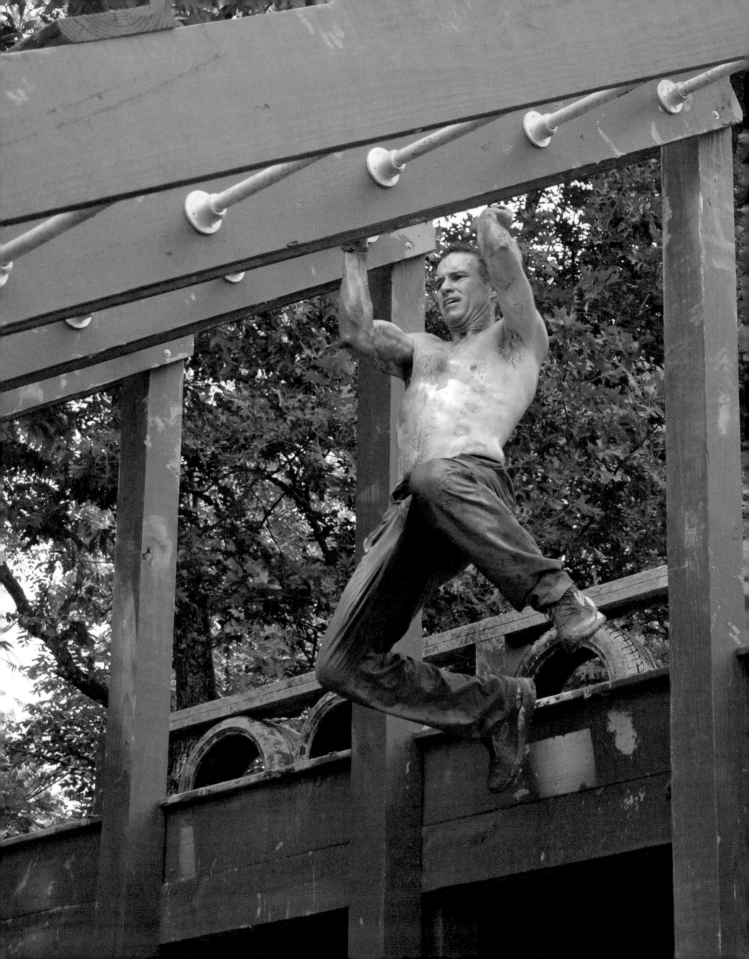

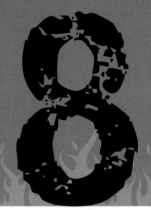

MASTERING THE MONKEY BARS

⚑ Featuring gymnast Anthony Matesi

I chose Anthony Matesi to contribute to this chapter because he's a former martial artist, gymnast, collegiate cheerleader, and now elite obstacle course racer. He placed third at the 2013 Alpha Warrior obstacle race in Southern California.

⚑ ⚑ ⚑

The monkey bars are a staple at almost every obstacle race course. Some are very straightforward and resemble the ones you jumped on as a kid. Others are far more difficult because the race creators have slanted them and inverted them over large pits of water.

Increasing Your Strength

To understand how to train for the monkey bars, we first need to analyze the breakdown of the movements involved in conquering this obstacle, and then we'll talk about how to prepare the muscles. Start with the first point of contact with the obstacle: your hands. What do they do when traversing a monkey bars section? They grip the bar. You need grip strength, and with it, forearm strength.

Don't stop there, though. When you're swinging from bar to bar, your entire body is hanging there, being completely supported by your hands and arms. That means you need to work your biceps.

What else is being used the most when monkeying around? Your back. Those muscles—the traps, the lats, and the

◄ *Let's get you ready to conquer these.*

shoulders—are all being activated when you're going across the monkey bars. So that's where our focus will be.

Let's start with grip strength. There are a variety of ways to work on this, but the simplest is to jump up on a bar and hang—for as long as you can. Then hang some more. You can time yourself to set a baseline. From there, work to continually improve the length of time that you can hang. This is a great progression to begin with if you are not capable of doing a pull-up at this stage of your fitness journey.

Once you begin doing pull-ups, I recommend adding in a dead hang at the end of sets to make sure you completely exhaust your hanging strength. Make it hurt but within reason. There's a difference between feeling exhausted and sore and risking injury. Be aware when pushing yourself past your boundaries.

Here are some other exercises you can do to strengthen your arms and back.

- Push-ups (regular, wide, diamond, etc.)
- Burpees
- Reverse dips
- Farmers carries
- Lat pull-downs
- Military presses
- Bicep curls (high, low, full, preacher)

- Rows (seated and upright)
- Tire flips
- Tire pulls and drags

The possibilities are endless. To work on your strength, your best option is to go to a playground. Find some monkey bars and get used to them. Swing from bar to bar. Hang for as long as you can. Test yourself.

Did your grip slip right away? If so, you need to toughen up your hands a bit. I do not recommend gloves. Build up calluses, and focus on improving the amount of time you can stay on the monkey bars without coming down.

An alternative option is working with a teammate to build up the ability to move from one monkey bar to the next. You'll want to have someone who is capable of helping to guide you across. Various methods can include sitting on your teammates shoulders, which does little for you. Or you can have your teammate simply bear hug your legs and help hold you as you traverse from one monkey bar to the next. As you become stronger, rely less and less on your friend's support to cross the monkey bars. Soon enough, you'll find yourself rockin' it out side by side.

Practicing Your Technique

There are a few different techniques you can use to conquer the monkey bars.

ONE AT A TIME: Many people will begin taking on the bars in a very controlled fashion. The athlete will begin by reaching up for the monkey bars and starting with both hands on the same bar. As the body comes to hang, one arm reaches for the next bar, taking hold as his fingers wrap around. Once the first hand is secure, the athlete releases the arm from the initial bar, joining his lead hand on the same bar. From there, the process is repeated, moving from one bar to the next, always rejoining both hands at each new bar. This method is slow and steady, but you can become faster as your strength, confidence, and grip improve.

APE SWING: With the ape swing, you start with one hand gripping the first monkey bar. You then reach your other arm for the next bar. Once your hand is gripping both bars, you let go with the back arm and swing your body forward, reaching for the next monkey bar and skipping the one that your other hand is still holding on to. Continue swinging from one bar to the next without bringing both hands onto the same bar

until you reach the very last one. Here, bring both hands to the last bar prior to dismounting.

HALF-PULL-UP/MUSCLE THROUGH: This technique requires you to have considerable strength. The idea behind this one is that you will hold yourself in a half-pull-up position the entire time you scale your way across the monkey bars. You'll need to be strong enough to perform this one, because you will not be utilizing the momentum of a swing to traverse from one bar to the next. While traversing, you will grab each bar with both hands like the one-at-a-time method, except the difference here is all about speed. You want to move fast

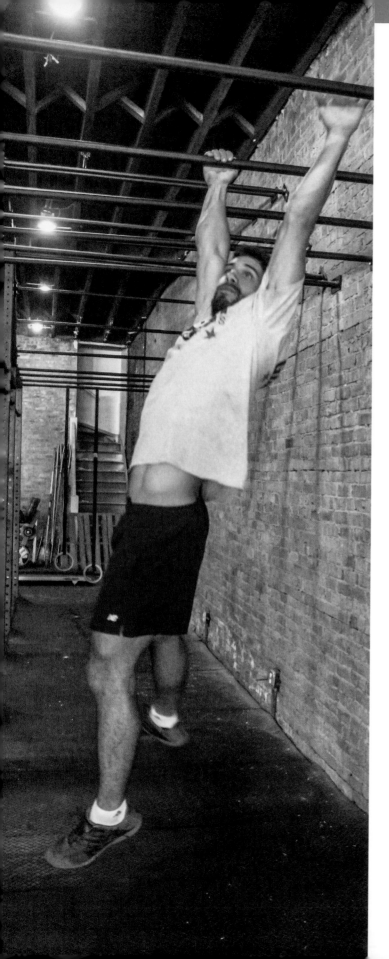

while holding yourself in the half-pull-up position. This technique is excellent for people who have recovered from shoulder injuries and have difficulty letting their body hang and swing. Another benefit to muscling through is a decreased chance of falling off due to slick hands from the water or mud you are likely to encounter before this obstacle at most OCRs with monkey bars. The reason for that is you have more control over regripping the bar should you start to slip. When you are holding on from a body hang, and your hand starts to slip, it takes more effort to catch yourself and readjust. Most of the time, once you start slipping from a full body hang, it's game over.

Race Day Tips

SKIP THE GLOVES. I already mentioned I don't recommend wearing gloves. Some people say they help, especially in the beginning when your hands are still soft and weak. However, in practice and at the races, it's common to find gloves tossed away within a few miles into the race. The mud tends to make the gloves slicker and actually inhibits the ability to complete many obstacles, including the rope climb, slippery wall, and the monkey bars.

◀ *Here Anthony Matesi demonstrates the ape swing method.*

I recommended experimenting with and without gloves before the race. Find what works best for you. The best option is to toughen your paws, work on building calluses, and increase your grip strength.

DRY YOUR HANDS. Often at races, you'll approach obstacles that are drenched and covered in muddy slop. Usually, you are also a slippery mess, and anything you grab is bound to slide out from your grip. If you're approaching an obstacle that requires your grip, such as the monkey bars or even the spear throw, look around and find something that you can use to wipe those slip-n-slide mitts dry. Tall grass and hay are often your best options. After you complete the obstacle, again dry your hands as quickly as possible.

CHECK BEFORE YOU TOUCH ANY-THING. Be careful and aware of what you're grabbing hold of. These races take place in nature, and that means there are many plants that you'll want to avoid grabbing, including but most definitely not limited to, poison ivy, oak, and sumac, stinging nettles, and thorn bushes galore. You don't want to become victim to itchy rashes or have to spend the night using a pair of tweezers.

TAKE THE CLEANEST PATH POSSIBLE. Many times when you approach an obstacle such as the monkey bars, there will be multiple lanes for competitors to keep the flow moving. Sometimes one set of bars will be cleaner or less used than others. It's wise to approach obstacles with an observant eye. Scan the bars, and opt for the ones with the least amount of filth, mud, and water on them.

As the day progresses, it's unlikely you'll find any clean sections on the bars. In these instances, look for the driest path you can find.

Don't let something you can fix prevent you from completing this obstacle. Always be on your toes when racing, aware of your surroundings, and conscious of the natural elements that can aid you in completing the race and conquering the obstacles.

Continue to Improve

Once the monkey bars become an obstacle of ease, remember that you can always improve. Try going back and forth across the monkey bars as many times as you can until you can't hold on any longer. Keep striving to push yourself farther, longer. Make your body become the ultimate monkey bar climbing machine.

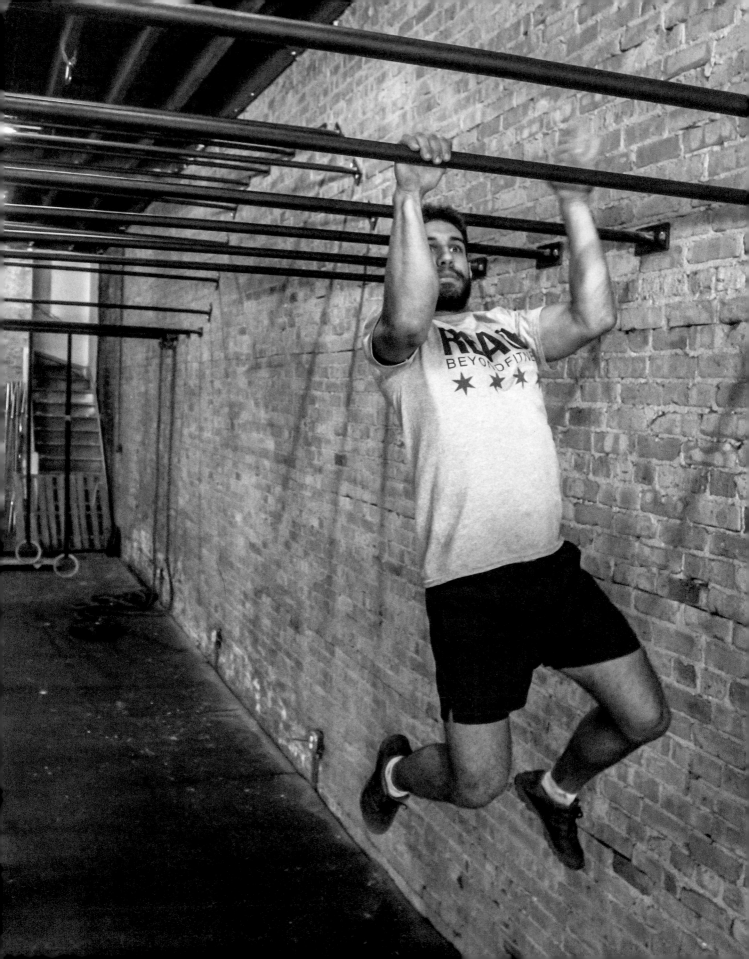

Always begin with establishing your baseline, go as far as you can, and take note of how many bars you did, or how many laps. Then try to go a little farther the next time. Or find incline and decline monkey bars, and practice on them. Challenge yourself to continually improve, and you can do great things.

Anthony Matesi is an entrepreneur, writer, and fitness coach at ReachBFC in Chicago. He's also a seasoned Death Race competitor and leads weekend excursions through his Legend of the Death Race Training Camps. Learn more at www.legendofthedeathrace.com.

DOWN AND DIRTY TAKEAWAYS

- **Hang in there.** Just hanging from a pull-up bar or monkey bars will start to build your grip strength and work key muscles specific to this obstacle. You can then move on to additional exercises.
- **Build calluses.** Some say gloves. I say no gloves.
- **Clean your hands off.** On race day, if you just came out of the mud, rub your hands in grass or dirt to make them less slippery.
- **Check obstacles prior to liftoff.** Choose monkey bars that are the driest and cleanest, if possible. If there is mud, look for dry, caked-on mud instead of wet mud.

◄ *The half pull-up.*

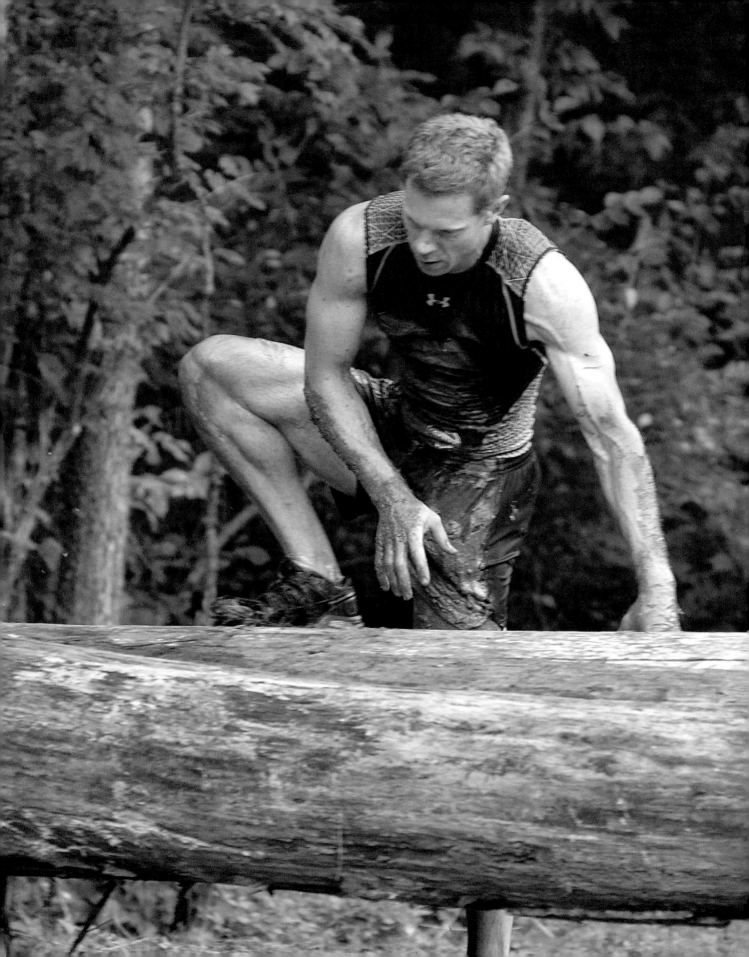

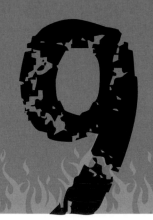

GETTING OVER WALLS AND OTHER OBSTACLES USING PARKOUR

✎ Featuring Parkour expert Matthew Willis

A mutual friend introduced me to Matthew Willis at the Texas Spartan Beast in December 2012. As we hopped the first short walls at that race, he let out the familiar (tongue-in-cheek) cry of "hard-core Parkour!" I began asking him lots of questions about the discipline of Parkour training, and I became fascinated with its applications to OCR.

◼ ◼ ◼

You may be wondering, "What is Parkour?" Or you might be thinking, "Wait, Parkour is that crazy French thing kids do when they jump off of buildings, bounce from wall to wall, and flip over stairs. How is that going to help me crawl through mud?" Good questions! Before I tell you whether or not Parkour can help you in an obstacle course race or not, I need to share with you a short history of Parkour.

A Brief History of Parkour

Parkour comes from the expression *parcours du combattant*, which loosely translates to "fighting the obstacles." The expression comes from the French military firefighter brigade, which often held competitions that involved overcoming obstacles quickly and efficiently. As those competitions continued, one male participant began to win over and over again. Raymond Belle took the concepts of Méthode Naturelle, which is a complete movement system with ten basic principles of movement, and applied it to his military firefighter brigade training.

◀ *Parkour movements can help you get over obstacles quickly and efficiently.*

The incredible ability that Belle possessed inspired his son, David Belle, to create something that was the opposite of the stringent and locked-down method of only ten principles, and take his newfound art to the streets of France: Parkour.

In the late 1980s, David Belle created Parkour and shared it with his friends and cousins. They began to explore more of the urban landscape and develop techniques that were more efficient for the common obstacles we have today. The movement of Parkour evolved over many years, and it has grown in popularity.

You can find a sprawling infrastructure of Parkour videos all over the Internet, and it's even featured in popular movies such as James Bond's *Casino Royale*.

Parkour in OCR

Now we can talk about how Parkour can help you in OCR. One way is by helping you use less energy as you overcome obstacles, and by allowing you to focus that extra energy on running, lifting, and carrying. Parkour is about efficiency of movement. Parkour is a tool that can help you more easily overcome obstacles. Next, we'll detail three direct ways Parkour training will help you in that next obstacle course race.

GET UP

Getting up a wall is one of the crowning achievements in an obstacle course race. Most racers are excited to come away from a wall having gotten over by themselves with relatively small amounts of bruises and torn-apart pride.

Using Parkour can help you get up and over those walls without spending the energy you need for running. Something that Parkour practitioners hang onto desperately is their technique. Most Parkour practitioners can climb up 10-foot (3-m) walls and drop right down from them without spending an exorbitant amount of strength, and repeat this process for hours. Deploying the right technique allows a practitioner with modest strength to outperform relatively stronger athletes. The following technique will help you to achieve a good wall scale—without having to rest on the other side of the wall.

"Parkour is about efficiency of movement."

1. Start with a good run up. Yes, you have to run at a wall, quite aggressively at that, too.

2. Once you get your forward momentum going, here comes another force of momentum. In Parkour, we call that

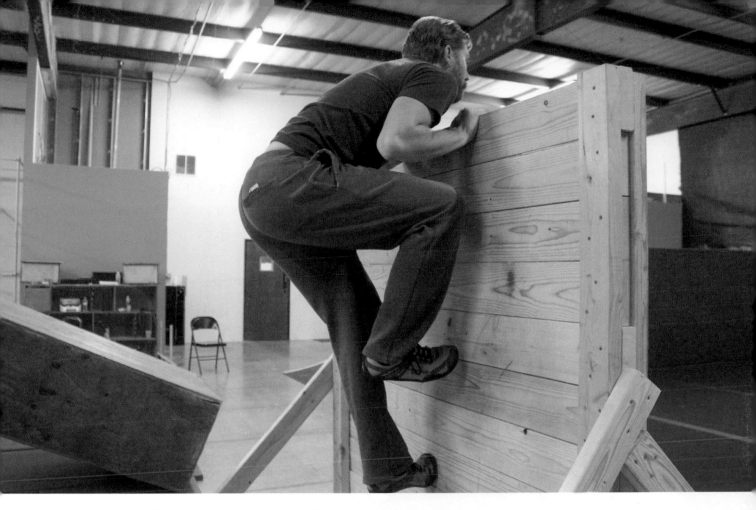

▲ *Don't stop your forward momentum when your foot hits the wall.*

force a "tac." That's using the ball of your foot to apply force into the wall at around hip height.

3. When forward momentum meets downward movement from your foot, you get lift off. Yes, you have mud on your foot, but this still allows for momentum up the wall and good positioning for climbing up and over that wall. Without getting your feet higher up on the wall, it will be hard to gain the right force of energy to overcome the obstacle.

4. While getting airborne, push all the way out of your foot to propel yourself upward. As you are tacing the wall, use that momentum to continue your hands to the top of the wall. OCRs generally have walls about 2 inches (5 cm) thick, so you should be able to get a significant amount of grip.

5. Now start pulling yourself up. Your momentum does not stop here in a hang. Use that momentum from your tac to continue pulling up the wall. If you think "pull" too late, you stop

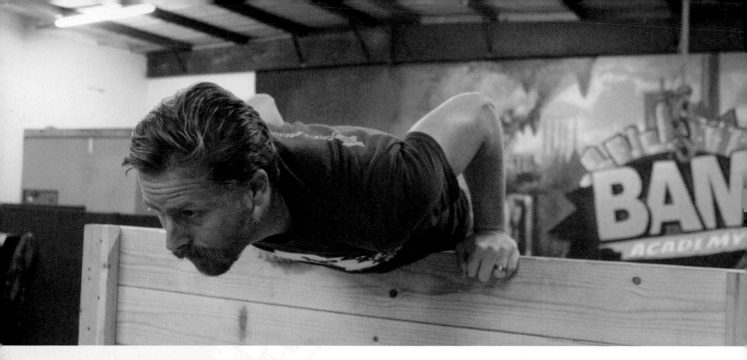

▲ *Pull yourself into the "beached whale" position, with your waist pulled up over the top of the wall.*

dead in your tracks and lose your speed up the wall; you will be stuck hanging, and your efficiency will be out the window. You should pull until getting into what we call the "beached whale" position, with your head hanging over the other side of the wall, then the wall pulled to your waist.

Pull your nose right over the top of the wall. Scrape your chest across the top of the wall. Keep your elbows in close to your body so that you don't spend any more energy than you have to with a wide-arm grip. Keep your body close to the wall. This allows you to do the most conservative pull-up, thus not spending extra energy. When overcoming these obstacles, you never want to be higher than you have to be.

6. Next, fight hard to get your upper chest over the wall. Use your feet to kick, climb, and scrape up the wall.

GET DOWN A SMALL WALL

Many racers think so much about getting up an obstacle that they might not even think about how getting down from an obstacle in a different way may increase your performance in a race. Using Parkour, you can jump from great heights or continue your momentum through obstacles with some simple techniques that are easily learned.

It's common to see racers jump over a 4-foot (1.2 m) wall with the greatest of ease, but then smash down into an "Iron Man" three-point stance on the other side of the wall. That should never be your

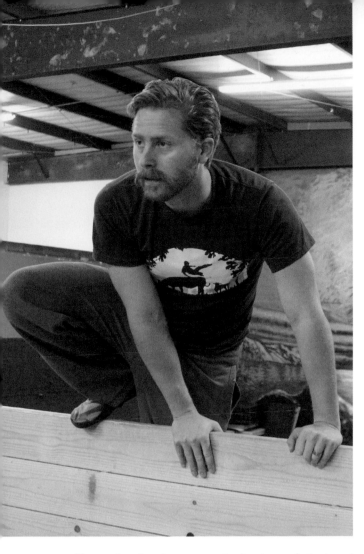

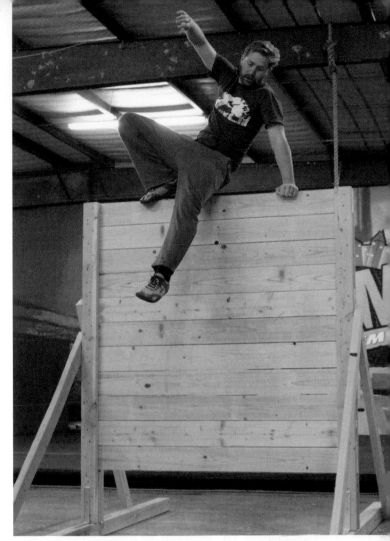

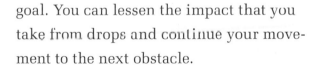
▲ Use one hand and your opposite foot to reach the top of the 4-foot wall.

▲ Bend your leg and arm to lower your hips and reduce the force with which you hit the ground.

goal. You can lessen the impact that you take from drops and continue your movement to the next obstacle.

1. When getting down from a low obstacle, such as a 4-foot (1.2 m) wall, you're going to find a way to vault or jump onto the obstacle. We are going to use a Parkour technique called the "safety down." It starts by bringing one hand and your opposite foot onto the top of the wall. When getting into this position, it's important to remember that your fingers should always be facing the direction you are going. This allows you to have the proper grip needed, and it gives you the force you need to keep your momentum moving forward. Your second leg is dangling in front of the obstacle waiting to strike the ground.

2. Next, lower yourself down from the obstacle. Bend your opposite side leg and arm to allow your hips to move lower beneath the top of the obstacle. From any height, lowering yourself down will allow you to save a harder strike on the ground.

3. After lowering yourself down from the obstacle, push away from the obstacle and use your other leg to reach onto your toes to step onto the ground.

4. Then use your opposite foot to continue on into your run. You can do this quite quickly and efficiently by trying to keep your momentum through the whole movement.

GET DOWN A TALL WALL

Your biggest waste of energy, however, is jumping from the top of 6-, 8-, and 10-foot (1.8 , 2.4 , and 3 m) walls. You want to find ways to lower yourself quickly without losing time and energy. When you learn the get-down technique that many Parkour practitioners use, you'll feel less like the wall is an obstacle and more of a way to shave minutes off your run while spending less energy.

1. Remember to keep your chest close to the wall. You want to drop your chest to the left or the right on top of the wall. One at a time, swing your legs over and bring yourself into a beached whale position. If you try to drop down from the wall from the top of the wall, you still have a chance of expending a lot of energy, tiring yourself for more obstacles to come.

2. While in a beached whale position, bend your first leg, sticking your foot to the wall. (Without your first leg sticking to the wall, you are very likely to just slide down the wall; this is why we bend that leg.)

3. Slowly lower yourself down the wall, keeping your foot against the wall and push, regulating your descent. After lowering, you will look just like you're doing your tac up the wall and reaching for the top.

4. Make sure to push away from the wall with your foot and land on your midfoot, allowing your legs to sink and absorb the shock of the fall. Don't bend your legs beyond a 90° angle. Going below 90° is not efficient because it allows for deep tissue exertion and unnecessary impact on your joints and tendons.

You could ask, "Why not just slide down the wall?" You could slide down the wall on the other side, however, lowering yourself in this way allows you to

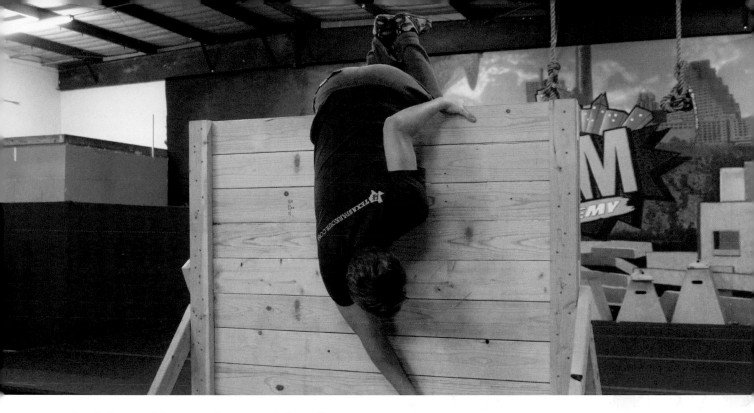

▲ *Reach down and drop your chest to touch the wall.*

stay in control of your movement. It keeps you from falling over the side, banging your knees or tearing up those ankles and heels while dropping. Often when sliding, however, you will fall close to the wall, and you have to bend your legs to absorb shock. When your legs bend, it will send your knees straight into the wall.

GATE VAULT

If you'd like to make getting down even more efficient, here's a final technique that will remind you more of a cartwheel than getting down a wall. It's very efficient and the fastest way of overcoming a wall.

1. Start in a beached whale position. Turn one hand so your fingers are pointing backward on top of the wall, and reach as far as you can down the wall you have just overcome and let your chest drop all the way until it's touching this side of the wall.

2. Pull hard on your hand turned backward, and push hard on your hand reaching, then pull your legs up and over the top of the wall on the side in which your arm is reaching. Pulling your legs on the opposite side will result in a cluster of flailing arms and legs to the ground. When performing this movement correctly, it will look more like a cartwheel over the wall than a drop off the wall. The most important part of this whole movement

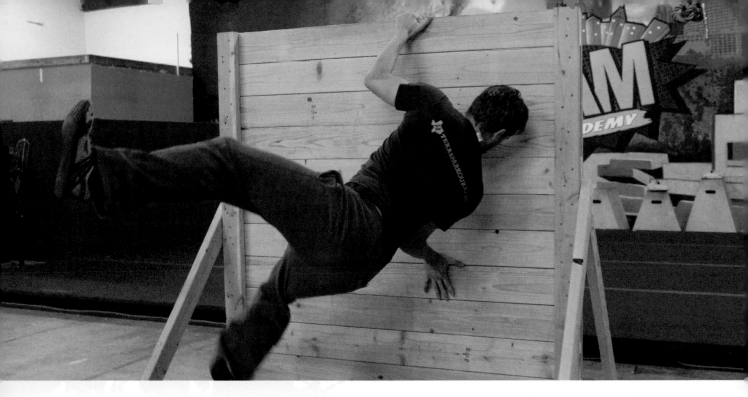

▲ *Keep your eyes on your lower hand as you bring your legs over and to the ground, completing your cartwheel.*

is that you keep your eyes on the hand reaching down on the wall. If you do not keep looking at your reaching hand, you are more likely to do a front flip than you are a cartwheel.

3. Now that you are pushing your legs up and over the wall, keep your arms holding strong, and try as efficiently as possible to bring your legs over to the ground one at a time. Your top hand will need to release once you get closer to the ground, or you will end up back into the wall.

4. Finishing this movement, you can push away from the wall cartwheeling out into a run. Cartwheeling out is the very last step and requires that you

twist your body, turning away from the obstacle at the last moment. However, starting out, you may practice by coming straight down over the wall, feet together while holding strong to the wall, landing near the wall.

This movement is potentially dangerous without a lot of training and practice, but this a fast and efficient movement that fits into Parkour because it allows you to continue your movement without having to stop for an obstacle. You must remember overall that jumping down from a wall spends too much energy and is a potential injury waiting to happen. You want to keep your legs healthy and strain-free.

GET OVER

Sometimes getting over something is the least of your problems in an obstacle course race. Like the linebackers that we think we are, we just barrel through obstacles—not worrying about clipping ankles, knees, or the people next to us. However, Parkour practitioners tend to think of movement in arcs rather than straight lines. Often people may think a straight line is the most efficient, but in Parkour, we find that if we treat obstacles in straight lines, we often spend too much energy trying to overcome them.

Let's take the dreaded balancing act as an example: the Log Hop. Although seen in several different arrangements, the Log Hop is generally made with telephone-pole-size logs sticking vertically out of the ground in a row, with several other logs to accompany. The point is to hop from log to log—up to 10 to 15 at a time—without hitting the ground and getting those dreaded burpees penalties.

"Parkour practitioners tend to think of movement in arcs rather than straight lines."

In Parkour, you follow your paths without hesitation, and you must keep your forward momentum—not for an instant thinking about moving backward or sideways or staying stationary. In Parkour, we employ a method called "striding." This is the act of hopping large distances, one foot at a time, onto obstacles and objects using our constant forward momentum. We use striding so that we do not spend precious energy hopping from log to log one at a time and stopping or using the dreaded contortion act of the "reaching across method," which usually results in an increased chance of injury or failure.

Striding subscribes to parabolic motion. Parabolic motion is like a rainbow, where we strive to jump up, across, and then finally down in the shape of a rainbow. So even though Parkour is seen as a straight line, arcs or parabolic motion are required to obtain maximum safety and assurance of success. Using the Log Hop as an example, this is how you would use Parkour to your advantage.

1. Try to wipe as much mud off the bottom of your shoes as possible before starting! However, you are mostly employing the toes of your shoes and do not require as much of the heels if done correctly.

2. Lean forward on the beginning log, and start driving your reaching leg's knee up while pushing hard out of the toes of your opposite leg. Pulling your

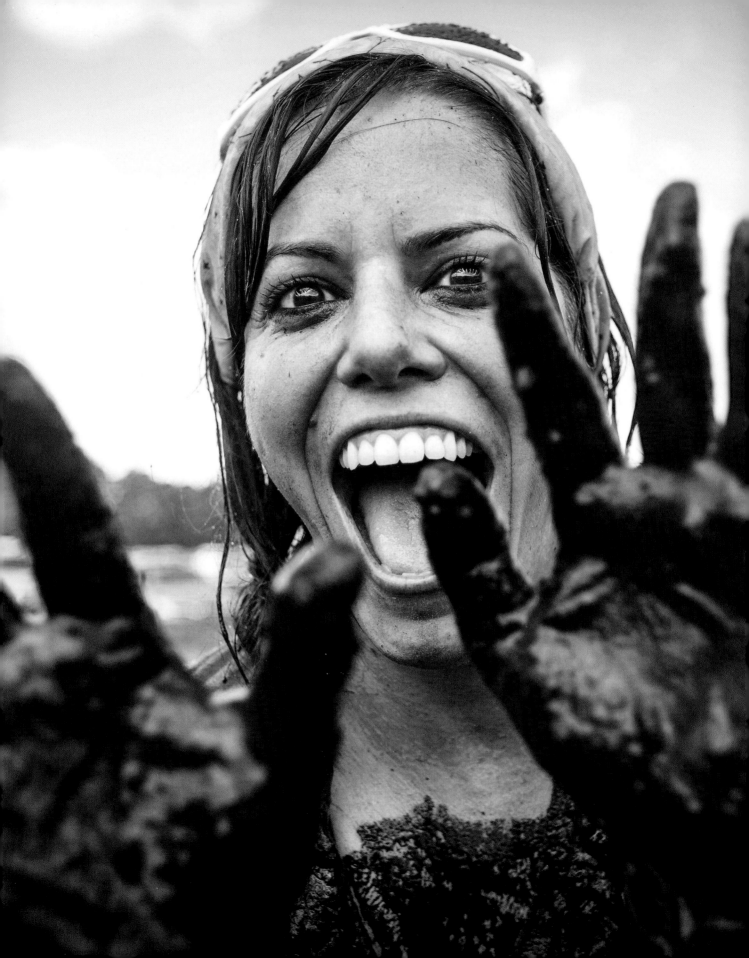

"reaching leg" up will help you get the parabolic motion that you require. It is not enough that you push forward and reach; you must get your weight up and in the air instead of driving in only one direction—forward. If you drive forward, there is generally enough mud and momentum on your feet that for the most part, it will be hard to stop and may result in slipping off the object.

3. As your arc begins to descend, you now have ample time to concentrate on the precise landing that you require to continue your motion. You want to land on the toe pad and not the heel of the foot. We are often less precise with the heel, and the heel will cause you to concentrate too much weight in one spot. Also, if you land on your heel, it will not allow your momentum to continue to reach forward with your toes so that you may continue onto your next jump. Instead, it will act more like a brake on a car, keeping you from moving forward.

4. Upon landing, you must absorb the impact from propelling your body up and down while bringing your next knee into the air, instantly ready for your next obstacle. Even though you are striding, it is halfway between a squat and a plyometric drill. Your body does not spring instantly from the object, but it allows you just enough time to absorb, judge, and redirect your energy to the next obstacle. It is important that you do not lower your body more than a slight knee bend to absorb your landing so that you can keep your momentum going forward. Too large of a knee bend will also result in loss of momentum and keep you from continuing your stride.

Striding can be extremely rewarding, though very difficult. One drill to use in training is to place cones or draw lines on the ground to practice this technique without too much punishment at first. You can often find poles at parks, universities, or playgrounds to get a better training regimen. When moving on to practice on something with height, just practice one pole at a time. You can start striding from one to another and getting to the point that your momentum continues, then move on to two and three poles until finally, your balance and coordination is enough to do it over and over again without hesitation.

◀ *Look, Ma! No hands!*

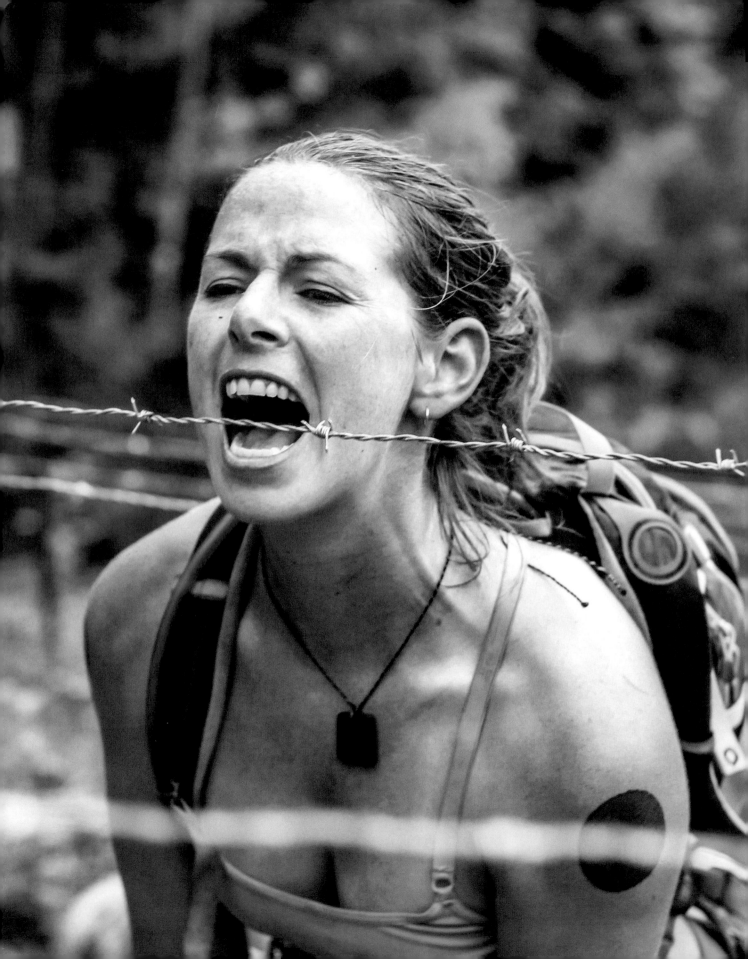

Parkour was created to help people get through obstacles better and faster. With these techniques, you'll find ways to adapt this movement to even more obstacles in the obstacle course world. With Parkour training and practical use of the discipline, you'll find ways to make the obstacles less about "if" you can tackle them, and more about using your body in a way that will break down less and have more energy.

In our obstacle course races, we have a competitive spirit, and we get in the zone. With adrenaline and our willingness to perform, we must minimize our risk of unknown injuries during a race. In races, you can sprain joints, tear tendons, and bruise limbs pretty badly and still run without too much understanding of the severity of the the injury. Using techniques like this saves you strength and allows you to get through the race injury-free. Parkour is going to help you accomplish your obstacle course racing goals—safely.

DOWN AND DIRTY TAKEAWAYS

- **Use efficiency of movement.** When you use less energy to overcome obstacles, you can focus that unused energy toward other things you will have to do in OCR, such as running, lifting, and carrying.
- **Learn to tac.** A proper tac shoots you up the wall to your highest point. It conserves more leg energy than leaping does.
- **Beach yourself on the way up.** The beached whale position conserves loads of arm energy.
- **Lessen your impact on the way down.** Learn ways to lower yourself that require much less energy.
- **Learn to stride.** When doing the Log Hop or similar obstacle, forward momentum is the key. When you start and stop, you're more likely to lose balance. The techniques in this chapter can help you master this.

As a second-generation Parkour athlete, Matthew Willis learned, trained, and taught with the originators of the Parkour discipline. He's the founder and organizer of Texas Parkour, Parkour Federation, and co-owner of BAM Academy, a 7,500-square-foot (700 square m) Parkour gym in Austin, Texas. Visit them on the web at www.truenaturetraining.com.

◄ *This book may not prepare you to eat barbed wire.*

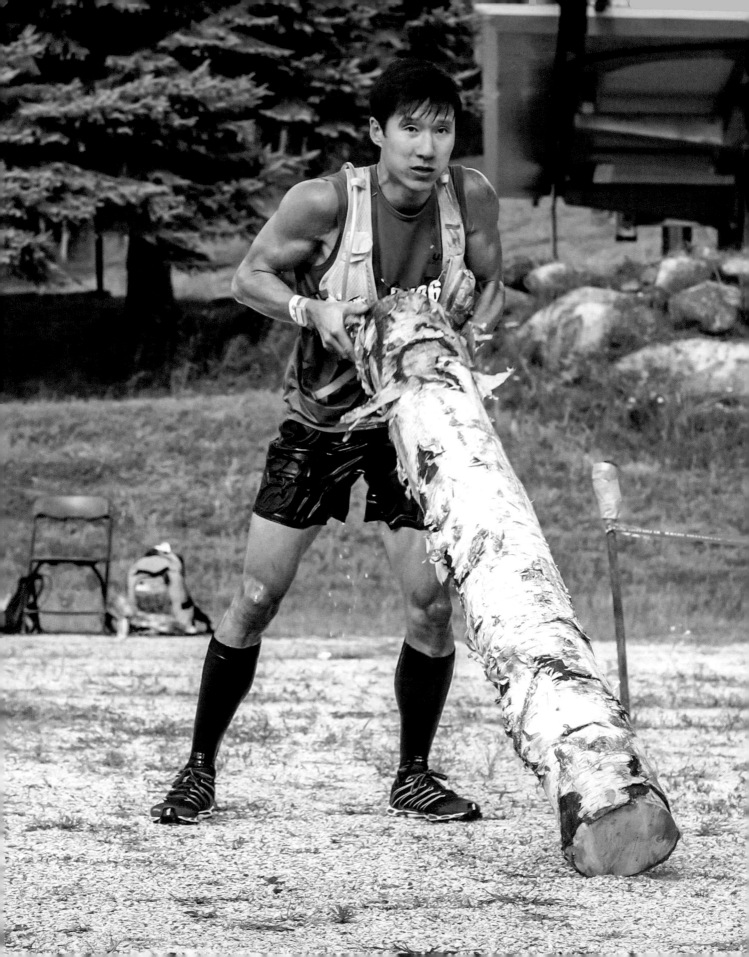

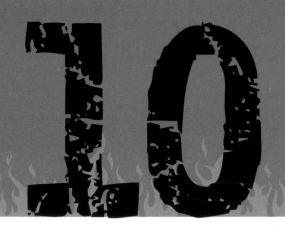

10 WORKING YOUR CORE

☙ Featuring obstacle coach Ekaterina "Solo" Solovieva

I have followed the writings of Ekaterina Solovieva a.k.a. "Solo" for a while. As an athlete and college professor, she consistently writes well-thought-out and well-researched stories on OCR. She also uses a wide variety of training techniques that help her stay in top physical form.

※ ※ ※

"Wow, you are hard core!" I hear from yet another friend who looks through endless pictures of me in the mud, under barbed wire, carrying things, dragging things, lifting things, and running for hours.

Why, yes. Yes, I am hard core. To be more accurate, I *have* a hard core. A strong core is incredibly important in the sport of obstacle course racing.

The common question that I get from racers is to how to strengthen the lower back. "Why the lower back?" I wonder. "Because I always feel it after the race," sighs yet another obstacle course racer friend.

❝Yes, I am hard core. To be more accurate, I *have* a hard core.❞

While seemingly unrelated, a sore lower back after physical exertion, be it a tough workout or a race, is a common symptom of a weak core. In fact, lower back pain is the second most common neurological condition reported in the United States, second only to headaches, according to the National Institute of Neurological Disorders and Stroke.

◀ *Having a strong core will help with almost every obstacle.*

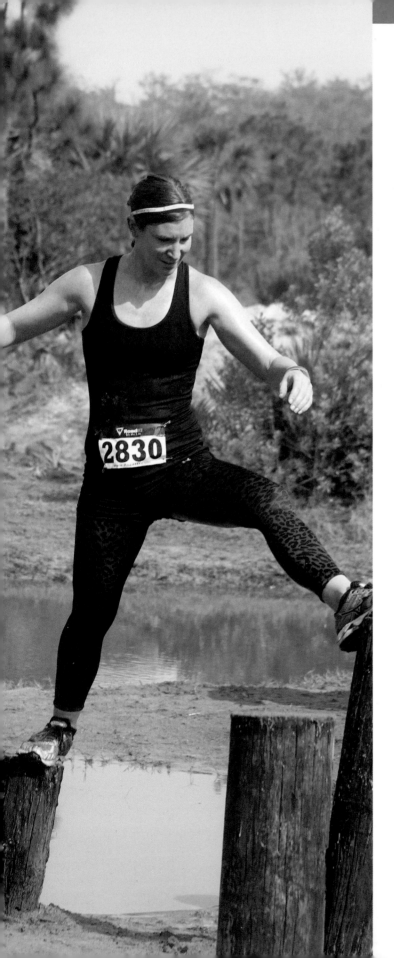

This is hardly surprising, given our sedentary lifestyles. Chances are good that even if you train and race regularly, a large portion of your day is spent in front of a screen with your shoulders hunched forward and your stomach relaxed.

Your Core Basics

Let's start at the beginning.

A "core" is the central part of a galaxy. The innermost part of something. The seed. The base. The essence.

Your core does not end with your stomach. "Core" refers to a wide band of muscles all around the torso, connecting your upper body to your lower body. Thus, strengthening the core will include strengthening the front, sides, and back. As a result of strengthening your core, you will improve your breathing, stability, and balance, and you will also prevent injury while running obstacle races.

In fact, some yogis believe that toning the abdominal region is a sure way to develop your inner strength as well. Is there anything a strong core cannot do?

Did you know core muscles are used during forced breathing? As your breathing becomes more labored, as it does during vigorous exercise, your body starts

◀ *Any movement that will challenge your balance will also strengthen your core.*

to engage more of the abdominal muscles with every inhalation and exhalation. Try breathing out forcefully, and you'll notice your stomach contract.

The transverse abdominis muscle, the deepest layer of the abdominal wall, contracts during forced exhalation, while intercostal muscles help to lift the ribs as you inhale.

For example, singing teachers will encourage their students to strengthen their core in order to improve their breathing. While you may not be singing the opera anytime soon, better breathing translates into more oxygen for the muscles, and therefore, better performance.

The Importance of Stability

Stability refers to your ability to hold your trunk steady as you move. Hitting a tennis ball, running down the track, or performing a deadlift all require a stable position of the body.

When do we need stability in an obstacle race? The perfect example is walking uphill. While it seems that your legs are doing all the work, a strong posture helps to keep you upright.

Obstacle race directors love hills. So you have to prepare for them. If you live near some mountains, get out and hike up and down them. If you don't live near

actual mountains, be sure to climb every single incline in the neighborhood time and time again. As racers get tired, their form suffers. They collapse through the middle and overload their lower backs.

Regular hill training will increase your speed both on flat and hilly surfaces. It will also be beneficial in conditioning both the legs and the core.

While the research findings regarding core stability training are mixed, it seems that incorporating core training into resistance training is especially effective. Exercise balls provide an easy way to include an unstable base into your workouts and to engage the core.

The Importance of Balance

When was the last time you had a balance workout? I thought so. We don't usually think about our balance until we lose it, and we're on our way to a face plant.

"Incorporating core training into resistance training is especially effective."

The vestibular system is the sensory system in your body that provides you with sense of balance and spatial orientation. Obstacles challenging your balance are appearing more and more often in the

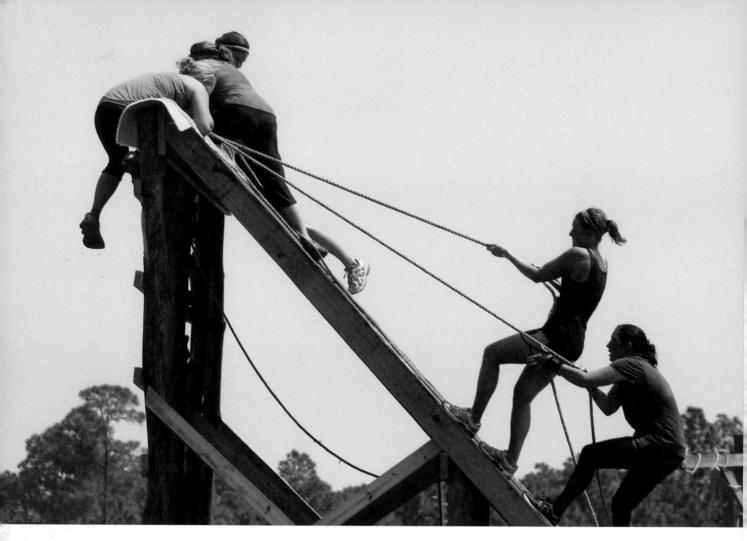

▲ *A strong core can prevent injury.*

sport. For example, participants have to traverse thin planks suspended in the air, jump over hurdles, or walk across a rotating log.

To improve your balance, try experiencing positions other than simply standing upright. Consider jumping, climbing, hanging upside down, and standing on your head. Try hopping onto a log next time you're running on a trail. Or try performing a familiar exercise, such as a shoulder press, while balancing on one leg. Try the yoga Tree Pose, balancing on one foot, while placing the sole of your other foot against the inner thigh of the standing leg.

Still too easy? Close your eyes. In addition to the vestibular system, visual input plays an important role in proprioception, the sense of your relative position in space. Removing the sense of vision severely impairs your ability to maintain an upright posture, and therefore, provides an excellent training opportunity.

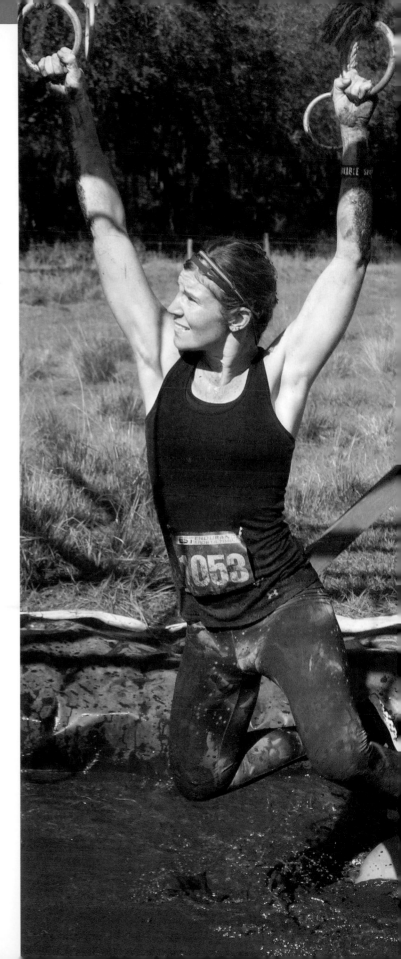

Preventing Injury

Having a strong core can help you to prevent an injury for two reasons.

First, a strong core can protect you if you fall. Falls are one of the leading causes of unintentional injuries in the United States, according to the National Safety Council. Slipping on a muddy downhill or falling off a rope climb or monkey bars are also some of the most common causes of injuries in obstacle racing.

Chiropractors and doctors often recommend strengthening the core as a way to minimize the chances of "slip and fall" injuries. If you lose your footing, regaining your balance will require a fast reaction time combined with the ability of the muscles to quickly take the unexpected load of the body weight. As the body braces for impact, the core muscles must engage. If these muscles are weak, injury may occur.

Second, having a strong core can help you to prevent an injury because your core will protect your lower back when completing obstacles. A strong abdominal region will allow you to carry those sandbags and cement stones without straining the relatively weaker lower back. When picking up a heavy weight, remember to

▶ *Strengthen that core to help you become "lord of the rings."*

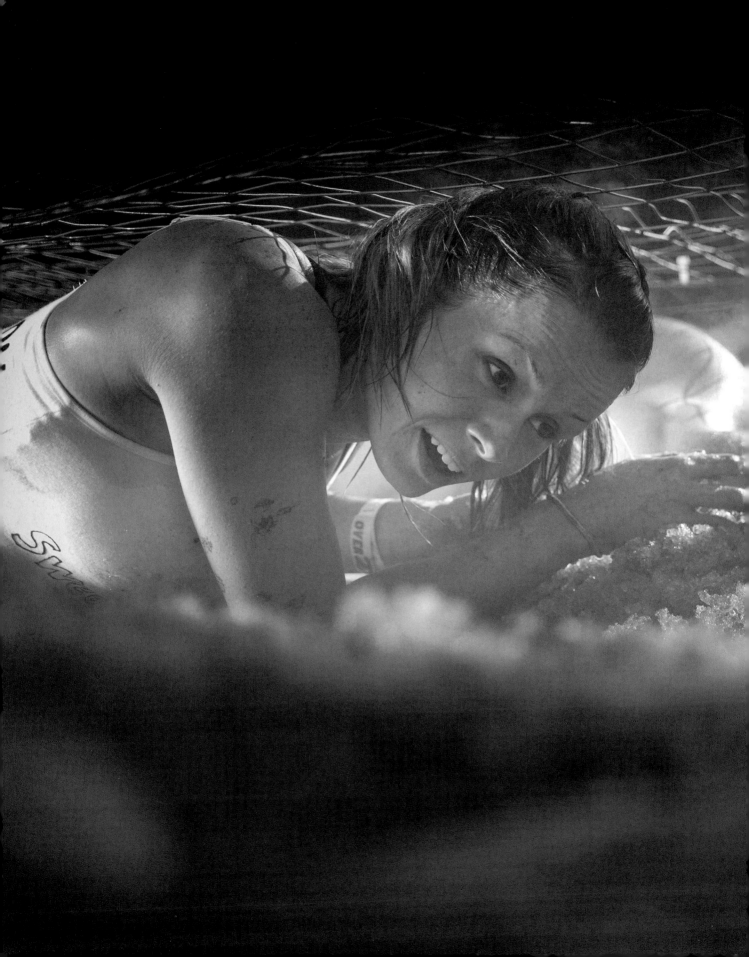

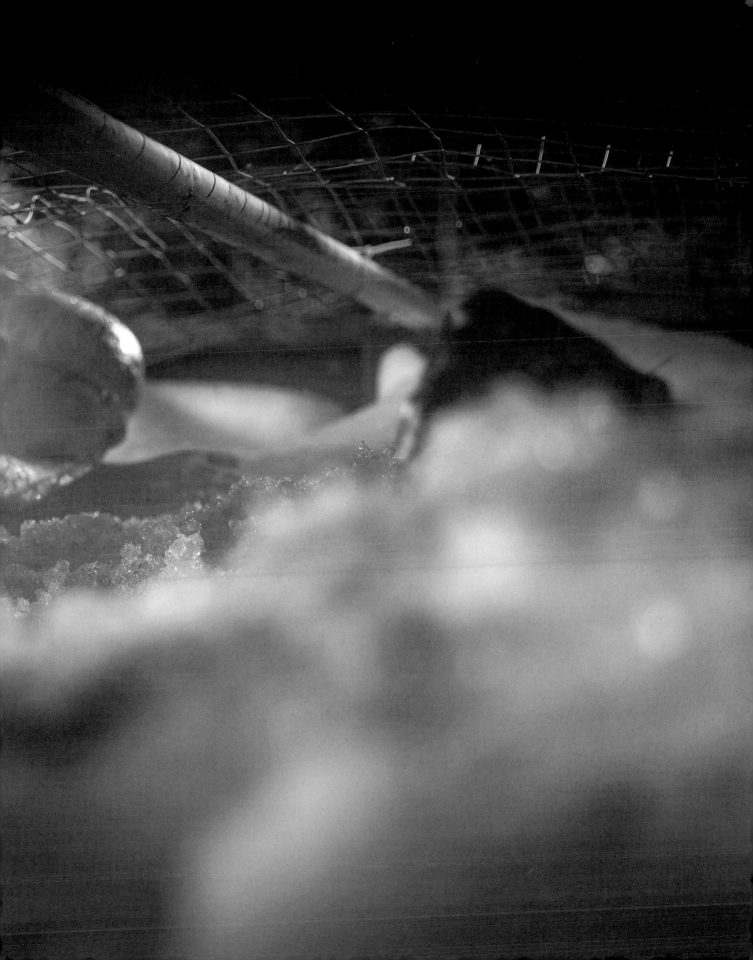

bend at the knees, as if you were doing a squat, keeping the hips flexed, core engaged, and back flat, then cradle the weight in your arms, and lift, using the legs.

How to Strengthen Your Core

Why don't I first tell you how *not* to strengthen your core? Don't do crunches. Please. For me. While it is possible to perform crunches safely, most of us simply lack the necessary body awareness required to do so.

Imagine the most shredded set of abs that you can find. I bet that if you approached their owner and asked if he/she did crunches, you'd get laughter in response. Even when performed correctly, crunches and sit-ups isolate the surface muscles, and they don't include the whole body. Instead of doing crunches, you need to include full-body compound movements in your training regimen. That will result in a strong, defined abdominal region.

It's important to note that you should do the bulk of your strengthening during the off-season. Racing season may not be the best time to start building strength.

Thankfully, there are many alternative ways of strengthening the core without straining the neck. Essentially, any exercise that will challenge your balance will also strengthen your core. Some examples include unstable planks on your side or with one leg up and one arm out, balancing your elbows on an exercise ball, or trying to balance a water bottle on the small of your back.

Consider exploring other activities and sports that will challenge your core. Often, simply changing up your usual training routine will be enough to discover the abdominal muscles you did not know you had. Belly dancing will introduce constant movement and hip figure eights as you focus on engaging the smaller core muscles. Yoga class will keep you sweaty with endless planks and balancing postures. And kickboxing will test your abdominal endurance and stability with quick jabs and knee thrusts.

In obstacle racing, the focus is on functional strength, rather than appearance. We're less concerned with getting "ripped" and more concerned with developing a core that's strong enough to support your body through any obstacle course race, be it a 12-mile (19.3 km) Tough Mudder or a 3-mile (4.8 km) Warrior Dash.

▶ *This is one you don't see at every race.*

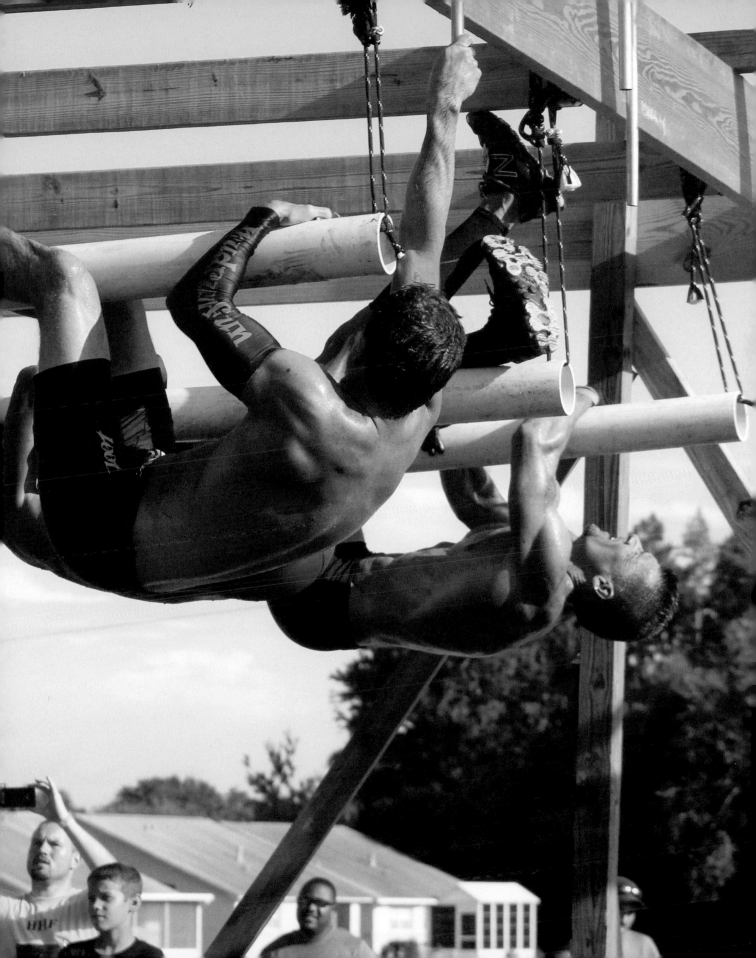

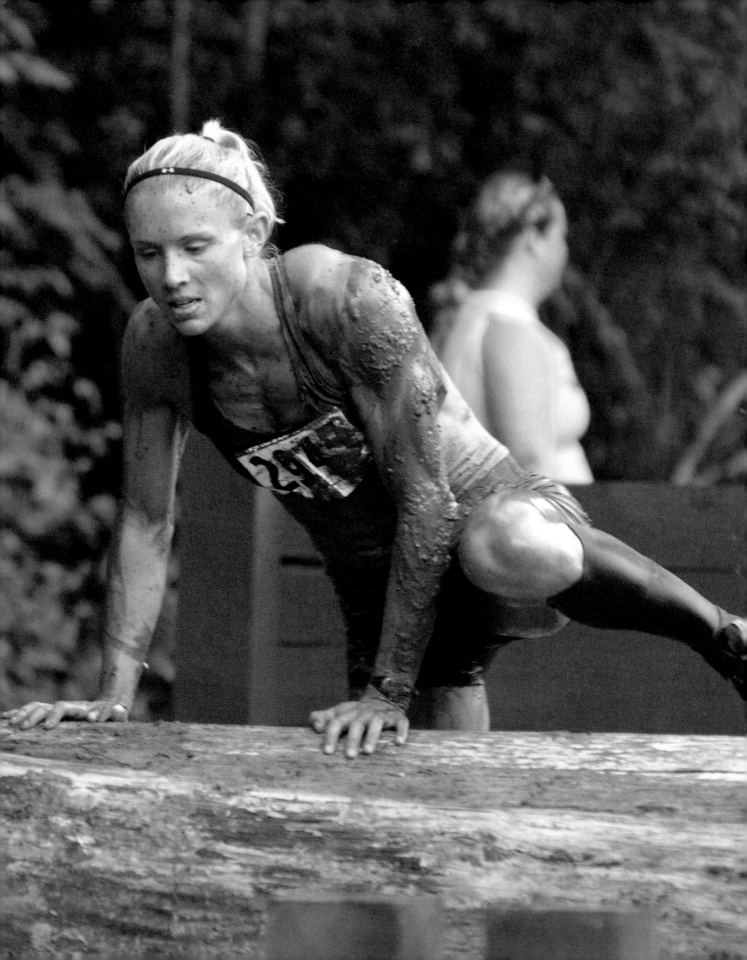

In your pursuit of a hard core, do not neglect other components of training. A good example of this is Bruce Lee. One of the most influential martial artists of all time, Lee was renowned for including all the elements of fitness into his training: strength, endurance, and flexibility.

Another way to look at it is to think of functional training, which originates in the field of rehabilitation. Functional training prepares the body to excel in the activities of daily life. Physical therapists working with patients include exercises that mimic what the patients will face at home or work.

> "Functional training prepares the body to excel in the activities of daily life."

Similarly, we need to consider what we may face on the obstacle course and train accordingly. For example, relative strength to your own body weight will be much more beneficial in an obstacle course race than absolute strength. It's much more helpful to be able to easily pull yourself over a fence than to bench press 200 pounds (90 kg).

DOWN AND DIRTY TAKEAWAYS

- **Learn to love hills.** Running up and down hills will improve your stability and increase your leg and core strength.
- **Challenge your balance.** Hop on logs and walk on the tops of walls. Do planks and other exercises that challenge your balance. Closing your eyes really makes you work for it.
- **Don't do crunches.** Forget what you read in the 1980s.
- **Train outside the box.** Do something outside the norm. Yoga, kickboxing, and belly dancing all work your core tremendously.

I'd like to leave you with a quote from Bruce Lee himself. Both in a race and in life, "Take things as they are. Punch when you have to punch. Kick when you have to kick."

Ekaterina "Solo" Solovieva is a Toronto, Canada–based obstacle course racer, health coach, and college professor. She writes about the sport of obstacle course racing, awesome gear, and all things extreme at www.solovieva.com.

◀ *Elite racer Amelia Boone has a really strong core.*

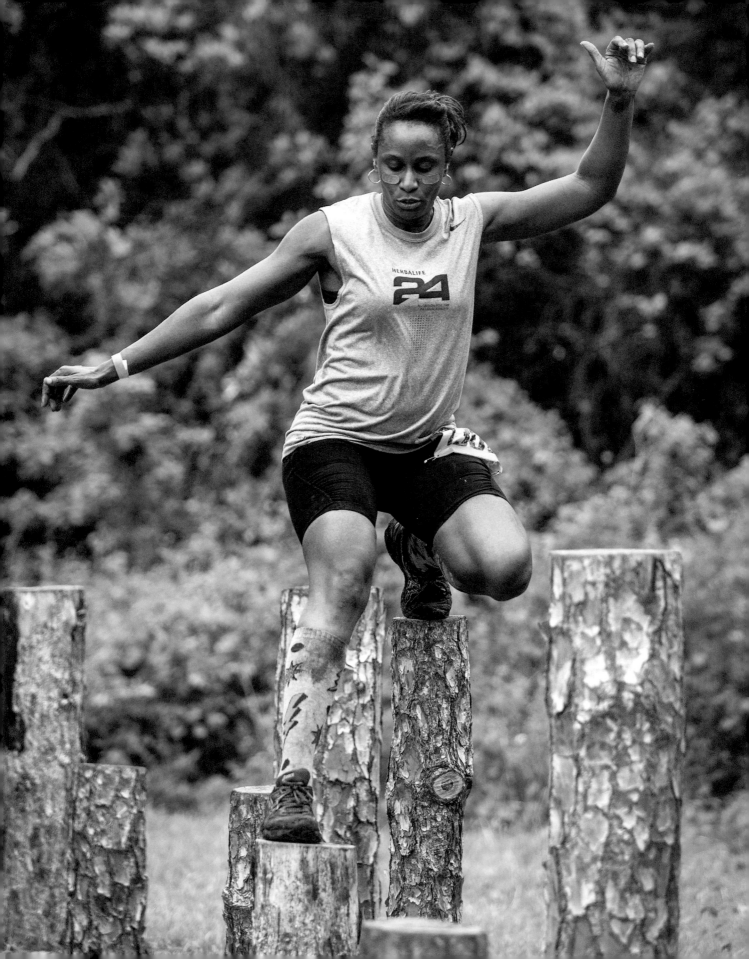

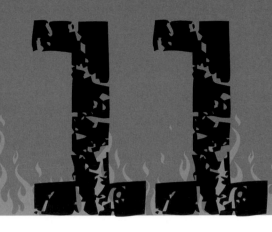

11 DOING PLYOMETRICS TRAINING

✒ Featuring Jeff Cain, EdD

After spending some time with Jeff and his wife (who he commonly refers to as "Mrs. on the way to Sparta") at a race earlier this year, I asked him to contribute a chapter on something that he knows a lot about, plyometrics, and that I felt could greatly help the OCR community as a whole.

※ ※ ※

I remember one sprint distance obstacle race early in my racing career in which I was struggling to keep pace with the guy in front of me. He had caught my attention before the race because he was wearing neon green running shorts and a sunshine yellow racing singlet with some witty running slogan on it. We were roughly the same size except that he was slightly more muscular than I was. He was fast. In fact, as we approached the first rolling mud hole obstacle, I had all but conceded that he was going to finish in front of me. Then something happened. He leaped over the mud hole. Actually, he tried to leap over it, but he came up a few inches short and splashed muddy water in every direction as he landed in the slushy hole. I jumped, landed steadily with both feet on the other side, scrambled up the berm, and continued on. I didn't see him again until after the race was over. He came sprinting in several minutes after me. As I reflect back on that race, I can't help but think that my jumping ability propelled me to finish in front of him.

I'm not naturally a gifted jumper. I've spent a considerable amount of time suffering through various plyometric workouts to be better.

◄ *Your plyo practice will pay off at the Log Hop.*

Plyometrics Basics

You may be asking yourself "What the heck is plyometrics?" It has nothing to do with that silly metric system that continues to confound American students. Plyometrics is often referred to as "jump training." It can involve any number of exercises that require repetitive, rapid stretching and contracting of muscles. Plyometric exercises are designed to create explosive and powerful movements, and they also condition the body for stable landings.

Plyo, as it is sometimes called, can be a useful component of any athlete's training arsenal. Relatively few sports don't require use of the fast-twitch muscle fibers that plyo targets. In fact, I can't even think of a single one at this moment.

"Plyometric exercises are designed to create explosive and powerful movements."

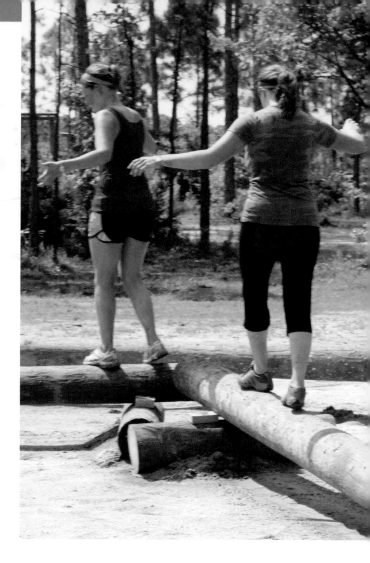

▲ *Plyometrics will increase your confidence and ability to bound up, over, and around obstacles quickly and easily.*

For purposes of obstacle course race training, why is plyo training important? Isn't running, cardio, and leg strength more important? Of course you should focus on those areas of fitness, but plyo will contribute to each of them. In addition to conditioning your body in a way that enables you to run faster, all the jumping and landing will help build the stabilizer muscles used for running. As for cardiovascular fitness, some plyo exercises are relatively easy, resulting in moderate elevations of heart rate. Others, however, will shoot the heart rate through the roof in a matter of seconds.

The ability to generate quick, explosive movements when reacting to changes in the course landscape is crucial for being fast on an obstacle course. Becoming good at plyometrics will increase your confidence and ability to bound up, over, and around obstacles quickly and easily. I can rattle off a long list of obstacles that plyo will help with. Obviously, jumping over anything will be enhanced: walls, logs, ditches, ravines, creeks, snakes, anything! You want to have the explosive ability necessary to propel you off the ground and up and over whatever stands in your path.

However, leaving the ground is not the sole act of jumping. You also have to come back down. That's when you need well-conditioned muscles that are accustomed to absorbing the impact of your body returning to earth. I cannot even count the number of times I have dropped from a wall, a rope, or a cargo net or jumped over a hole onto a muddy, uneven surface. Being able to land like a cat and spring away from potential ankle sprains is a valuable asset on an obstacle course.

A Brief History of Plyometrics

Believe it or not, plyometrics is not some new trendy fitness rage that has sprouted in the past few years. We all know about those. Can anyone say "Zumba?" Just teasing! Zumba is a great exercise routine, just not for obstacle racing. Don't hate me, Zumba people!

The term "plyometrics" was supposedly coined by an American track coach who observed the training routines of European Olympic athletes in the 1960s and 1970s. At that time, those athletes were dominating the sport of track and field.

For the anatomically minded, plyometrics involves rapid switching between concentric (while jumping) and eccentric (while landing) muscle contractions. Purists will insist that true plyometrics always involves this "shock" method of quick switches between concentric and eccentric contractions of the muscles. One can jump around without actually doing plyometrics.

Scientific studies have shown that plyometric training has significant positive effects for runners. Runners who incorporate plyometrics into their routines see greater gains in running efficiency. Plyometrics has also been shown to increase speed through enhanced eccentric and concentric muscle contractions and by conditioning the central nervous system to respond faster for quick movements. In addition to the speed and power gains, increased stability is an important safeguard against injuries.

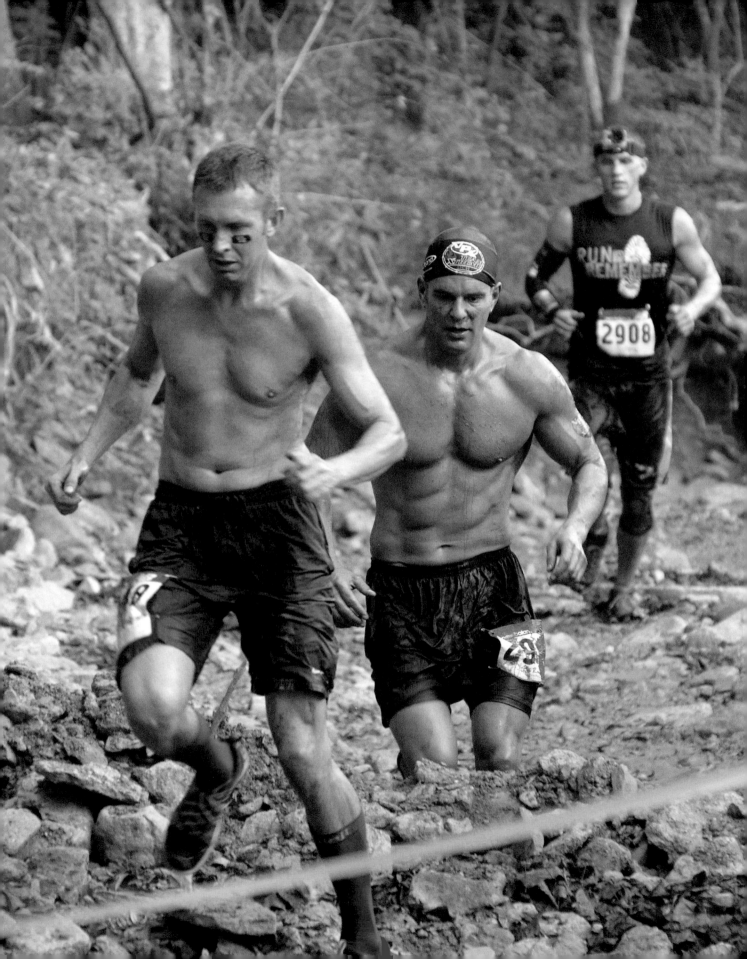

Trying Plyometrics

If you're just starting out with your exercise routine, don't go bananas with plyometric exercises. If your muscles, tendons, and connective tissues aren't ready for the rigors, there's a good chance that the injury bug will bite you. Ease into it. Just like any other exercise, you build strong muscles and connective tissue slowly over time.

I also feel obligated to offer additional words of caution. First, it should be obvious that if you have joint issues, weak ankles, or other medical concerns, you should consult with a sports medicine professional for guidance.

Assumedly though, you're reading this because of your interest in obstacle course racing. If your body isn't ready for plyometrics, it's a pretty safe bet that you're not ready for obstacle course racing. Put this book down, find yourself a good physical therapist, strengthen those weaknesses, and then come back to this chapter.

Here are some tips to get started.

CHOOSE THE RIGHT SURFACE. To avoid undue stress on your bones and joints, make sure the surface you use has some "give." Don't do plyo on a mattress, but absolutely don't attempt plyometrics on concrete or asphalt. Those surfaces are unforgiving and will likely cause serious damage to your body over the long term. Level grassy or dirt surfaces, mulch, or running tracks are ideal. If you're inside, use an exercise mat. The last thing you want from exercising is an injury that could have easily been avoided with an inexpensive mat purchased at the local sporting goods store.

WEAR THE PROPER FOOTWEAR. Some say that plyometrics is best done with bare feet; however, don't start out that way unless you're accustomed to going shoeless during exercise. Progress slowly. It's the rare person who can immediately withstand the force and trauma of jumps and landings on unprotected feet. Odds are that you're not that person.

On the other hand, avoid wearing cushiony running shoes. It seems like that would be a good idea, but it's not. Stick to lightweight training shoes with thin soles that allow for proprioception. (That's one of my top-ten favorite words. It essentially refers to an awareness of the spatial orientation of your body.)

◄ *Dr. Jeff Cain leads two other competitors by practicing what he preaches.*

FOCUS AS MUCH ON THE LANDING AS YOU DO ON THE JUMPING. Keep your feet, knees, and shoulders aligned as much as possible and slightly flexed. Land lightly on the balls of your feet, not on your heels or toes. Mentally picture yourself landing while making as little noise as possible.

BE CAREFUL WITH EXERCISES THAT HAVE YOU BOUNDING FROM SIDE TO SIDE. Knees and ankles are much better suited to withstand the rigors of front-to-back movements.

BOUND OFF THE LANDING QUICKLY. Although you should concentrate on landing technique, come back off the landing as quickly as possible. The benefits in these exercises come from spending as little time as possible on the ground. Think "soft and quick." Be a cat.

AVOID PLYOMETRICS AS YOUR PRIMARY CONDITIONING ROUTINE. Yes, it's excellent for getting your cardio mojo going, but you're asking for injury if you try to perform these while tired. Your form will break down, leading to joint, muscle, or connective tissue failures.

TIME YOUR PLYOMETRICS WORKOUTS CAREFULLY. Plyometric workouts should be highly focused, not endurance-based. A good rule of thumb (although by no means standard) is to exercise for up to 30 seconds, and then incorporate light active recovery exercises for a few seconds before going again. This will vary among individuals according to fitness level and per exercise. You either must honestly judge how well you can maintain form, or you could enlist the services of a trainer to monitor that for you.

DON'T DO EXTENSIVE PLYOMETRICS EVERY DAY. Like any other training routine, the gains come from the rest days as the muscles, ligaments, and tendons work to repair the micro tears induced by exercise. Two to three times per week is plenty.

Can you do more and get away with it? Perhaps. Sooner or later though, overtraining, whether it's plyometrics, running, or lifting, will begin producing negative returns as your body weakens from the stress. Be smart!

▶ *Reacting to changes in the course landscape with quick, explosive movements is crucial for speed on the course.*

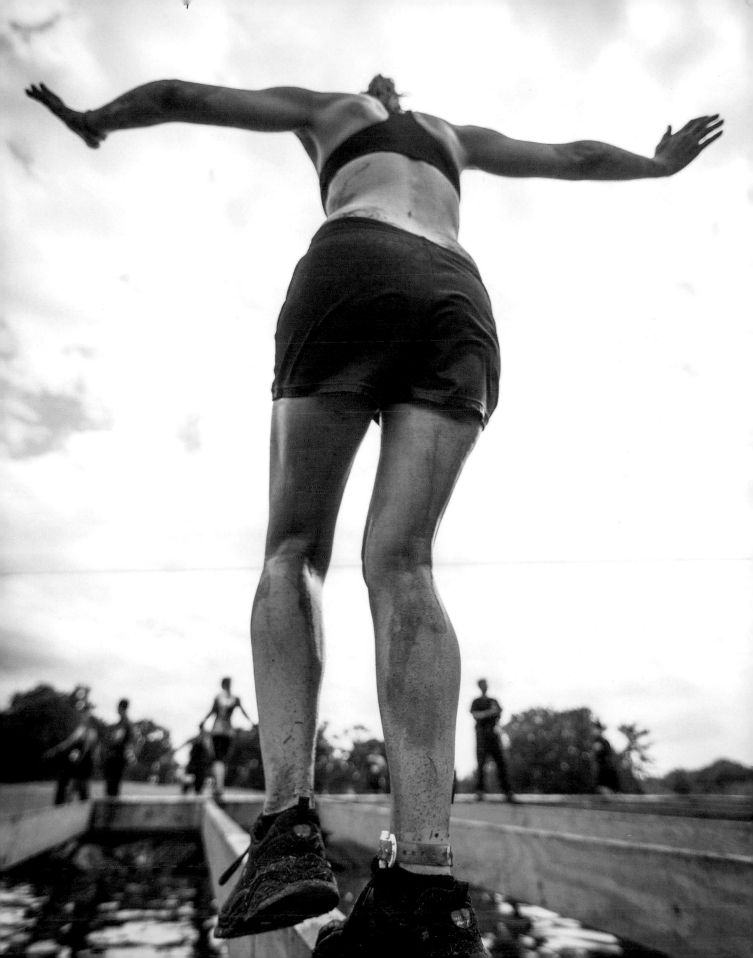

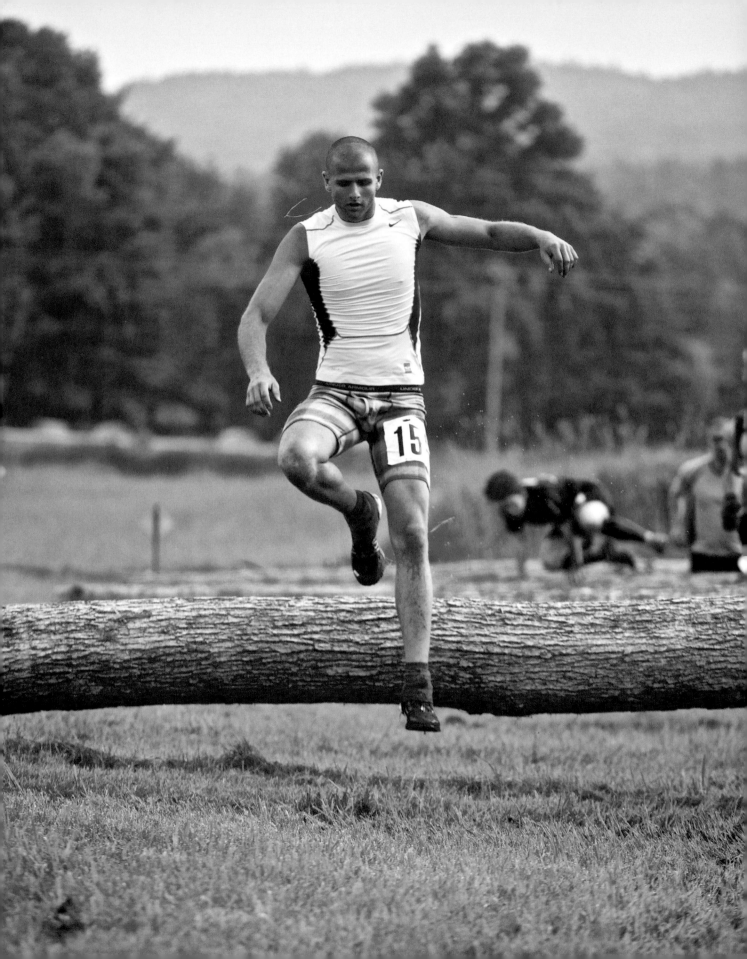

Plyometrics Basics

Plyo is easily worked into almost any exercise routine that you're currently doing. The exercises can range from very easy to extremely difficult, and anywhere along that continuum. Here are descriptions of various plyo exercises. These are just samples. You'll quickly learn that there are various modifications. The exercises are grouped into categories according to ease of performance. They can be combined for entire routines, or they can stand alone within other types of training. Personally, I will sometimes incorporate a set of plyo between weight or core exercises as a means of elevating my heart rate.

Always warm up before plyometrics. I spend at least 5 minutes warming up. The more time you spend getting loose, the better your workout will go.

Start with low-intensity movements that work the hips, legs, knees, and ankles, and then slowly increase in intensity. Standing knee raises followed by running in place is a good start. Slow and easy jumping jacks are a good second level. I usually end the warm-ups with active stretching exercises, such as leg swings (forward/backward and sideways), body-weight squats, and/or lunges. Ideally, you want your ankles, knees, and hips loose and ready for quick movements.

EASY PLYO EXERCISES

JUMP ROPE: At first, I had a lot of difficulty with jumping rope. Since I was a kid, I had always envisioned jumping rope as a little girl's exercise performed while chanting a silly cadence. That is until I watched the movie *Rocky*. It took me awhile to get the form down, but after rhythm has been established, it's easy to knock out 100 jumps. Because you don't have to jump very high, you may easily be able to do many more than 100. Jump for as long as you can, without sacrificing form. Quick jumps are better than slow ones. Keep your body aligned vertically from ankles, to knees, to hips, to shoulders, and land on the balls of your feet.

CROSS HOPS. This can be performed a variety of ways, but the simplest is to hop off both feet back and forth across and along the length of a line—which can be tape, a jump rope, or even a line drawn on the floor—for 8 to 10 feet (2.4 to 3 m), and

◄ *Being able to land like a cat and spring away from potential ankle sprains is a valuable skill in a race.*

then jump backward to the start. Repeat the process two or three times. Hop quickly and land softly. You can enhance this exercise by hopping higher and bringing your knees closer to your chest while still maintaining the same speed of bounding off the ground. Another variation of this is to hop side to side and back and forth. Or you could envision yourself jumping in the four quadrants of a large plus symbol.

MODERATE PLYO EXERCISES

SINGLE-LEG JUMP ROPE. Adequate enough description, right? Jump rope on one leg for 5 to 10 repetitions, switch to the other foot, and back and forth, for a total of 50 to 100 total reps. You'll find this much more stressful on the ankles and legs than regular jump ropes, so start at the low end of the range and work yourself up. Let your body be the guide on the amount of stress you can handle here.

SINGLE-LEG CROSS HOPS. This is just like the cross hops described earlier, except you hop with only one foot for 30 seconds or so, and then switch to the other foot.

DIFFICULT PLYO EXERCISES

JUMP KNEE TUCKS. Stand straight with your knees slightly bent and then jump by bringing your quadriceps parallel with the floor. Hold your hands out, with your forearms parallel to the floor to provide a target for how high you should jump. Land softly on the balls of your feet and immediately explode back up, bringing your knees back to your target. Perform 10 to 25 repetitions, depending on your ability. Don't sacrifice your form!

DOUBLE-UNDERS. A staple CrossFit exercise, double-unders are simply rope jumps in which the rope passes under your feet twice on each jump. This will send your heart rate to the max very quickly, so you won't need many reps. Start with ten at a time and work your way up to thirty. It's crucial that you maintain a good vertically aligned posture. If you start bending over, hunching, or generally just feel awkward, then stop, rest briefly, and start again.

BOX JUMPS. Another CrossFit exercise, this one is easy to describe. Start by standing in front of a stable box or other platform that is 18 to 30 inches (45 to 75 cm) off the ground. Jump onto the box. Land softly. Immediately jump back off the box and repeat as quickly as possible. You can do these for time (approximately

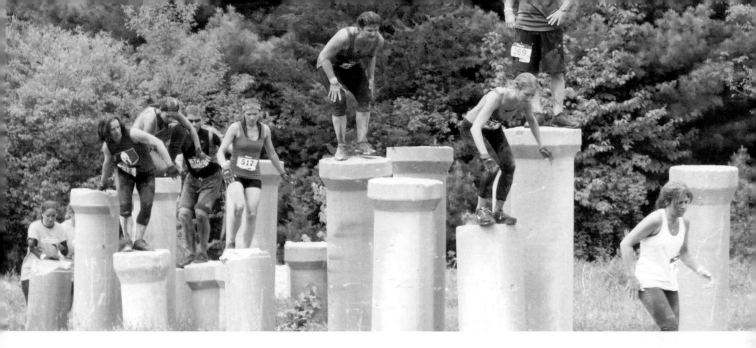

▲ *Good plyo exercises will have you master hopping obstacles like this one.*

20 to 30 seconds) or numbers of repetitions. Be careful with these. When form breaks down, you could find yourself losing a layer of skin (or worse) on the box edge.

JUMPING LUNGES. Put yourself in a slight lunge stance. Jump up and switch your legs so they land with the opposite leg in a lunge. Immediately repeat this. Ten of these will have you breathing heavily. Make sure you maintain good form.

Jeff Cain, EdD, is an obstacle racer and associate professor at the University of Kentucky College of Pharmacy. Follow his blog at www.onmywaytosparta.com.

DOWN AND DIRTY TAKEAWAYS

- **Exercise caution.** Always stretch first. Also, never perform plyo workouts on concrete.
- **Go minimal.** Minimal footwear or barefoot breeds the best results in plyometrics training. Avoid shoes with lots of cushion.
- **Don't overdo it.** Don't use plyo when you're tired.

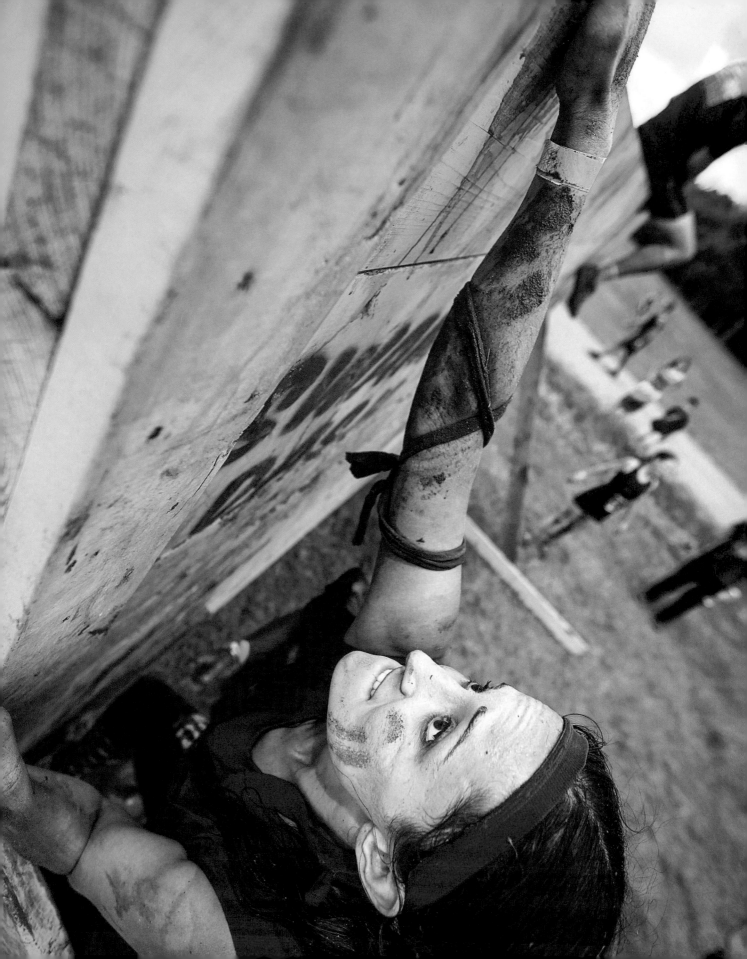

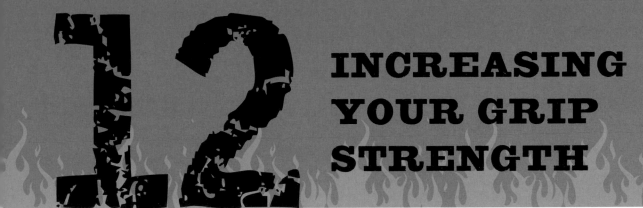

12 INCREASING YOUR GRIP STRENGTH

☙ Featuring obstacle builder Rob Butler

Rob Butler built the most difficult obstacles that I have ever come across at Shale Hill in Vermont. After I was tortured on his course, we had a conversation that led to this chapter. Grip strength is a much-needed, but often overlooked, part of functional fitness that can greatly improve your overall OCR performance.

❧ ❧ ❧

People often ask what makes someone a strong obstacle racer. Some people think it takes a strong runner, and others think you need strong arms and a strong core. These are all true, but if you can't hold yourself up with your hands, you can't finish an obstacle course race properly.

I believe that most people can get through the running end of an obstacle course race without too much trouble. Where most people fail is on obstacles that require a lot of grip strength.

I've had some success in generating a grip that works well for obstacle domination. Here are my quick tips for developing a gorilla-like grip—without really changing your workout schedule too much.

TRAIN YOUR HANDS FIRST. Many people think that by lifting more weights in the gym, their arms will be stronger, and therefore their hands will be stronger. This is not necessarily the case. A giant arm does you no good if you can't hold onto whatever you're grabbing. If you train the hand, the arm will follow.

◀ *You will need a strong grip for almost everything you encounter on the obstacle course.*

When you're using machines in the gym, try to replace any metal handles with ropes. Doing lat pull-downs, use ropes. Use cable machines for curls and use a rope. Do not allow your hands to touch the knots or rubber balls on the end of the ropes. Instead, use your grip.

When you're doing pull-ups, hang a rope or a rolled-up towel over a bar or beam and force yourself to use your grip in a vertical fashion. When you hold a pull-up bar with a hook grip, you're not really working the necessary muscles for rope climbing and general "hanging on" stuff.

Consider using a push-up pipe (PUP). I designed a product for Sinergy that was specifically made for the development of hand and wrist strength for obstacle course racing. It forces you to work all the tiny little muscles in your hands and wrists. These are the little muscles that will save you when you need to hold on to something for more than a couple of minutes, such as a Tarzan swing, rope climb, or traverse wall.

BUILD LONG, LEAN MUSCLES. In the gym, I never lift a lot of weight. Instead, I start with a small amount of weight and do hundreds of reps. This builds long, lean muscles, not large bulky ones. Here's why: The more nonfunctional muscle you build, the more weight you have to carry around the course with you. Often in an obstacle course race, you'll find really large dudes on the sidelines, dead tired from lugging around all of their weight.

TOUGHEN UP YOUR HANDS. One commonly overlooked aspect of grip strength is hand toughness. I have yet to find a pair of gloves that will protect your hands and work in all of the situations that obstacle course racing throws at you. I do everything bare handed: in the gym, on the training course, and in the races. One way to toughen your hands up is to simply climb ropes. Another technique I have used to build toughness as well as

> "I do everything bare handed: in the gym, on the training course, and in the races."

grip strength is to find a couple of small logs about 4 inches (10 cm) in diameter and 16 to 24 inches (40 to 61 cm) long with some rough bark on them. Carry these on your long runs, one in each hand. This will slowly toughen the skin

▶ *Lean muscle and great grip strength make a huge difference for this obstacle course racer.*

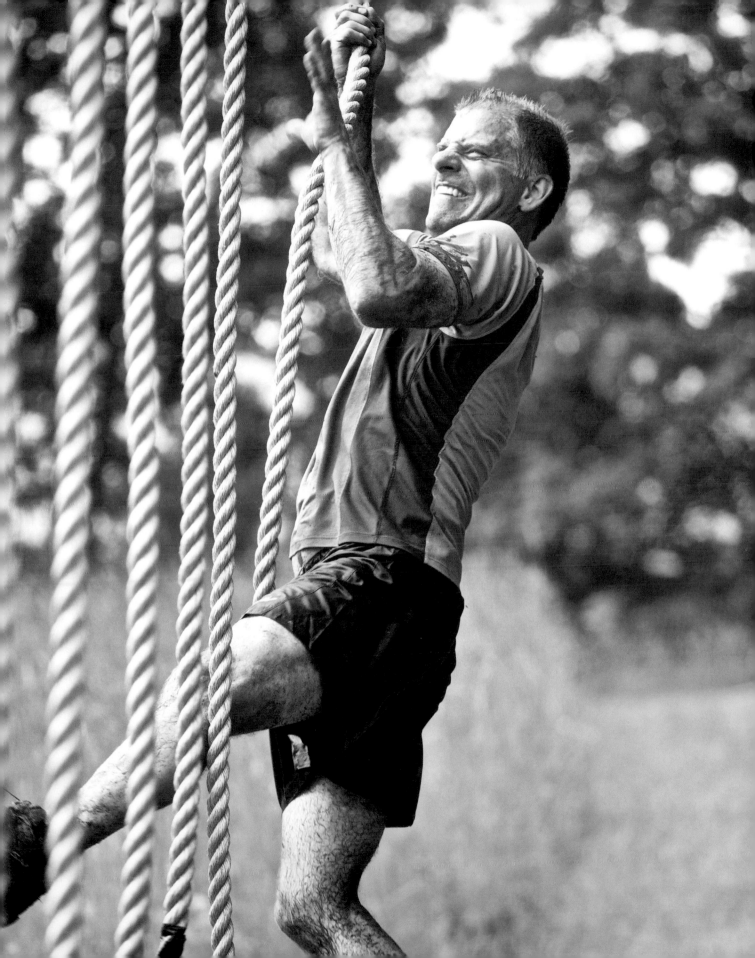

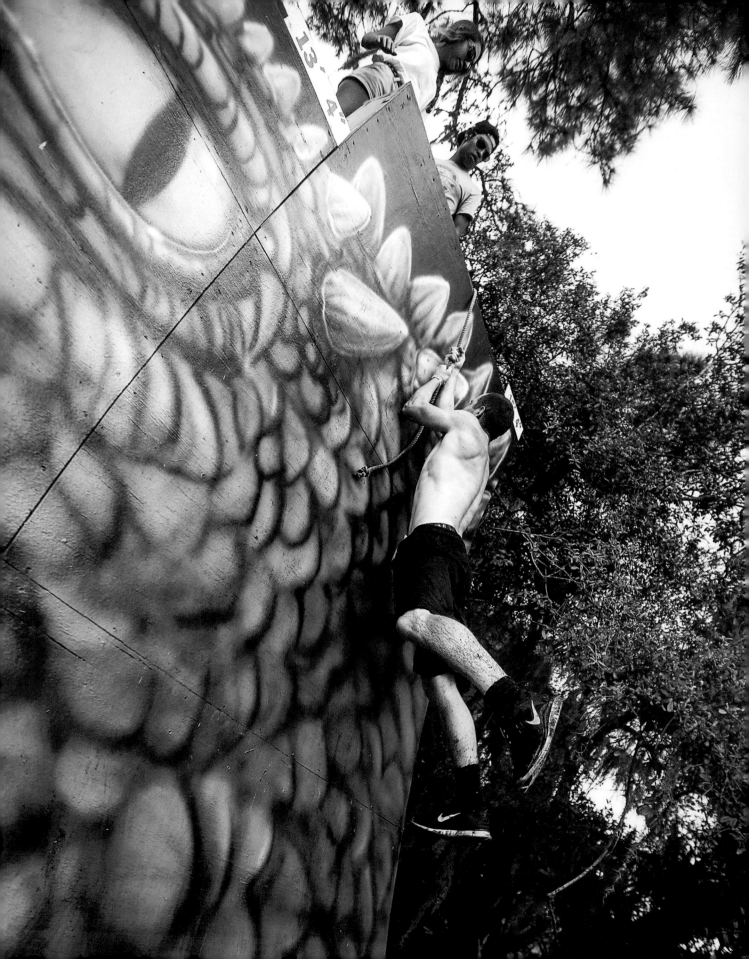

on your hands as well as get your body used to using your grip for a long period of time.

PRACTICE GOOD GRIP TECHNIQUE.
Another commonly overlooked aspect of grip strength is grip technique. When most people grab a rope, they simply put their hand around it and squeeze. To properly grip a rope or any other object in this sport, you must first wrap your fingers tightly around it and roll it tightly into the palm of your hand. This can be easily understood by simply opening your right hand, palm up, and taking your left index finger and placing it across all four fingers at the first joint down from your right-hand middle finger. Now simply close your fingers around the left hand pointer finger, locking into the palm of your hand right where your fingers are connected. Now pull all of your fingers into the palm of your hand and wrap your right thumb over your right index and middle finger. As you can see, you have generated two gripping mechanisms working together to supply a vice-like grip. The concept is the same with larger rope and trees and such.

With a strong, durable set of hands, obstacle training and racing will be much more enjoyable and rewarding!

Rob Butler has been constructing obstacles for the past three years. You can purchase OCR training equipment that Rob designs at www.sinergyobstacle.com. When in New England, please visit his one-of-a-kind training course and facility. Learn more about it at www.shalehilladventure.com.

◄ *With a strong, durable set of hands, obstacle training and racing will be much more enjoyable and rewarding.*

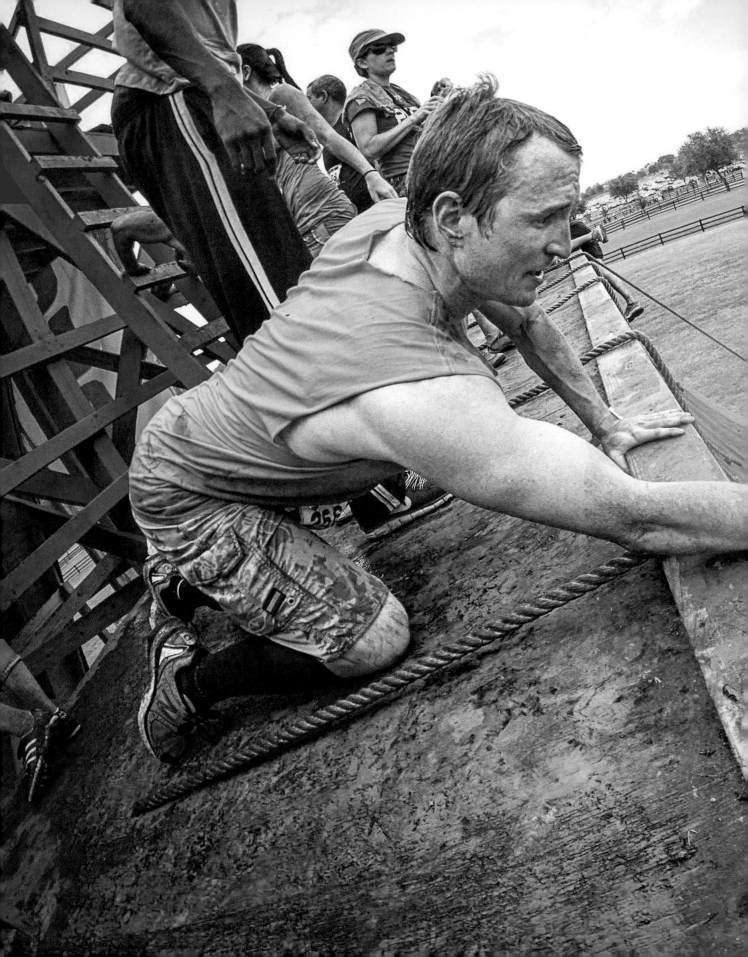

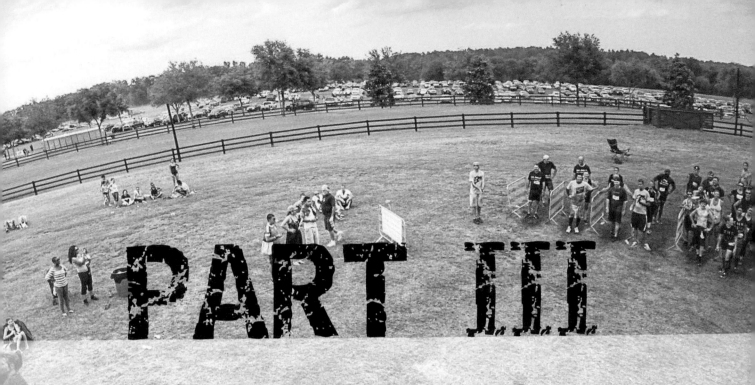

PART III

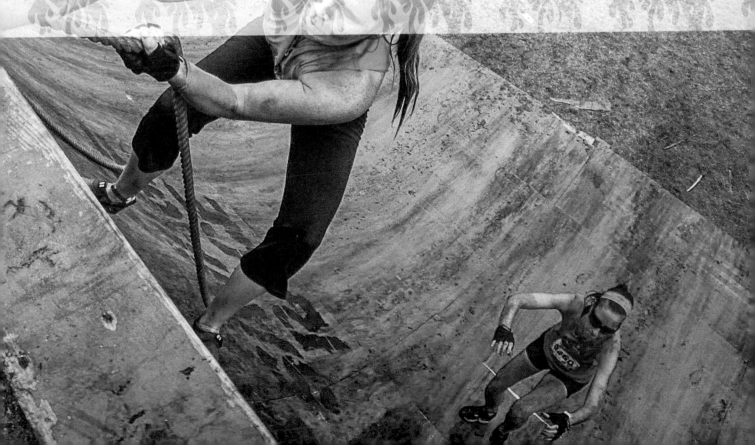

ADDITIONAL TOOLS
FOR MIND AND BODY

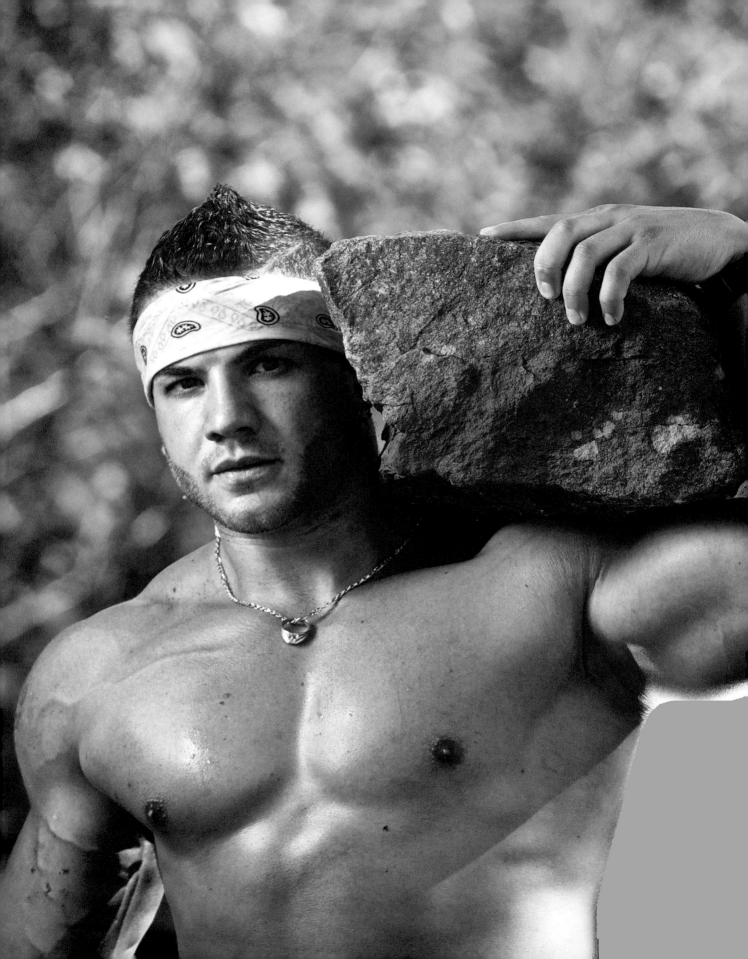

13 FINDING MOTIVATION

✒ Featuring Doug Grady

I met Doug Grady through another friend of mine, Dominic Carubba. Dominic is the once out-of-shape friend I referred to in chapter 7. (Dominic was going to sign up for a Tough Mudder, and my thought was, "If he can do it, I can do it." Doug was Dominic's roommate, and it was Doug's inspiration that got Dominic excited to sign up in the first place.)

Many months later, I began a friendship with Doug. I credit Doug with indirectly starting me on my new life and career in obstacle course racing. Prior to doing his first Tough Mudder, Doug was already a successful salesman, speaker, and motivator. He took those lifelong skills, along with the recent events in his life, to create something called "Muddervation."

✒ ✒ ✒

"When life gets muddy, get tough, my friend."
—*"The (unofficial) Tough Mudder Song"*

I find obstacle course racing a magnificent, muddy metaphor for life. On the path to your personal potential, there will be walls, roadblocks, and barriers of many kinds. Your relationship to these obstacles is a major factor in achieving at a high level.

"If you're going to achieve, there will be roadblocks. But obstacles don't have to stop you. If you run into a wall, don't turn around and give up. Figure out how to climb it, go through it, or work around it."
—*Michael Jordan*

◄ *Motivation comes in many forms.*

A few short years ago, I was stuck in the mud. I was out of shape, mentally dull, heavily in debt, emotionally unstable, and engaged in destructive tendencies. Just as success has a cycle, failure does as well. I was living it.

My turnaround began with a commitment to exercising a minimum of 30 minutes per day. Somewhere along the way, I registered for my first obstacle course race.

Registering had an immediate impact on my workouts. They became more interesting, purposeful, intense, and fun. Completing my OCR, which was much more challenging than I anticipated, opened up breakthroughs in every area of my life.

Many days, I just didn't feel like training. But I did it anyway. Feelings can be misleading. Do you know the hardest part about exercise for most people? It's not the physical act of working out. It's getting off your butt and getting to the gym, the trail, or even your floor. The pre-workout feelings often instill a sense that the task will be far more unpleasant, difficult, or tedious than it actually is.

I don't always feel like exercising, but I tend to feel good *after* a workout. You may not always feel like sticking with your commitments. You may not always feel like you're making progress. You may not always feel like doing the things you know you need to do. You may have to take your feelings out of it.

You may at times feel irritable, frustrated, agitated, overwhelmed, exasperated, confused, and befuddled. Do it anyway! Honoring your word feels good, and knowing you're making progress despite your "feelings" feels good. Hitting one of your major goals feels *fantastic!*

"Completing my OCR, which was much more challenging than I anticipated, opened up breakthroughs in every area of my life."

Success takes disciplined, consistent action over long periods of time.

Commitment has very little to do with feeling. Commitment means you do it anyway—whether you feel like it or not, whether it's easy or not, whether it's pleasant or not, whether you're too busy or not, whether you're tired or not, and whether it's convenient or not. When you consistently do what you say you are going to do, you develop confidence, inner strength, momentum, and, ultimately, character.

For me, it wasn't the training or even the completion of the challenge that made the biggest difference. It was paying attention to what showed up in my life as a result.

Each day, I forced myself to pay attention to the "ripples"—the progress, no matter how big or seemingly small, that emerged because of the shift in my lifestyle. I would notice and focus on my slightly better attitude, an increase in energy, or an unexpected, powerful conversation. I met extraordinary people along the way. I made other positive choices, which impacted my health, my business, and my relationships. I got stronger in my faith.

Positive choices are a great start. Showing up is a great start. Consistently honoring your choice is a great start. But it's just the beginning.

For maximum benefit to occur, it is not enough to simply do the work. You must pay attention to the positive results showing up in your life.

By now you may be asking, "How do I do this?" Great question. In fact, *questions are the answer*. Our awareness is determined by the questions we repeatedly ask ourselves. They tend to come in the following two categories.

DISEMPOWERING QUESTIONS
- Why is this so hard?
- How come I haven't made more progress?
- What am I doing wrong?
- Why do I keep having these problems?
- Why can't I do this?

EMPOWERING QUESTIONS
- What am I learning?
- How am I growing?
- What positive results have occurred because of the positive choice(s) I have made?
- How have my conversations been affected?
- How has my environment changed?
- What's different about my attitude and my energy?
- How have others been affected in a positive way?
- What am I grateful for?

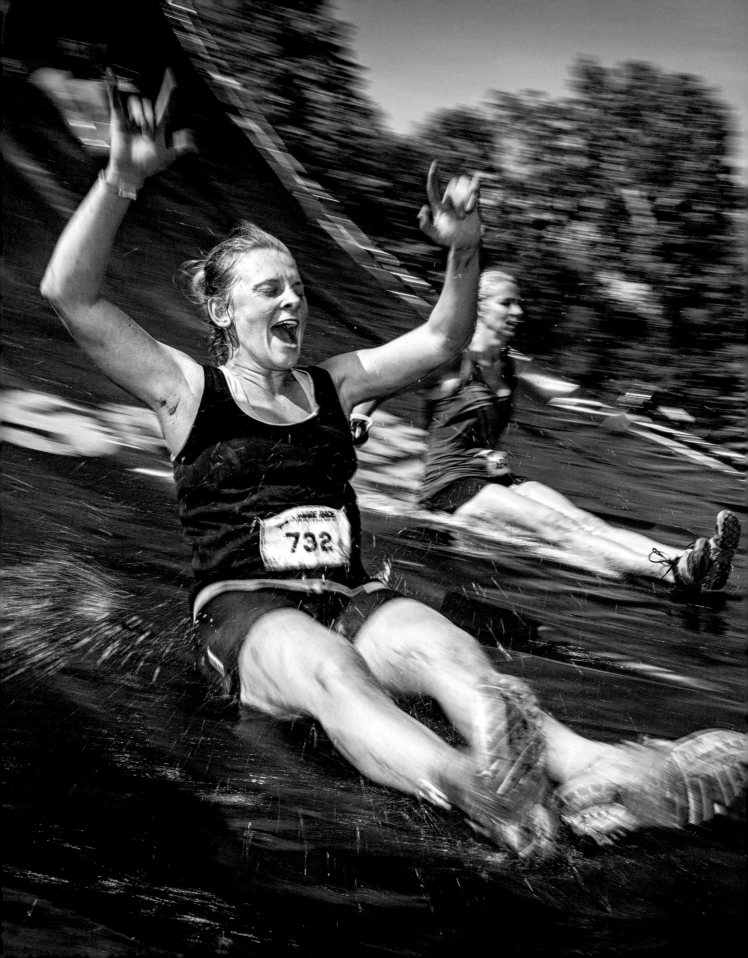

Become acutely aware of the positive impact your choices are generating. More positive choices will tend to follow. This develops momentum and increases the velocity at which you experience breakthroughs in every area of your life.

Motivating Exercises

Hint: They're not just for the gym.

BECOME AWARE. At least three times a day, become acutely aware of your thoughts. Personally, I do this first thing in the morning, during my daily workout, and at least one other time during the day. Like an outsider looking in, label them "empowering" or "disempowering." Don't beat yourself up for having disempowering thoughts. This is akin to feeling bad that you are feeling bad. Simply notice. What are the questions you ask yourself to generate these thoughts? Record this in a journal.

ASK BETTER QUESTIONS. Come up with at least six empowering questions and answer them daily, even if you have to force yourself. Record this in your journal or notebook. Pay attention to the answers, no matter how seemingly insignificant they may be.

CELEBRATE VICTORIES REGULARLY. Generally speaking, obstacles fall into two categories: external and internal.

External obstacles are outside of you. They include:

- Conditions; for example, I live in the wrong neighborhood, my car broke down, the cost of doing business is high, the weather is bad, the dog ate my homework

- Lack of resources, such as not enough money, time, equipment, education, or connections.

- Other people, such as the naysayer, unhealthy relationships, lack of family support, and poor role models

Internal obstacles lie within you. They include:

- Characteristics, such as race, sex, age, physical appearance, and background

- Physical limitations

- Beliefs; for example, I'm not good enough, smart enough, talented enough, or educated enough

- Negative emotions, such as fear, anger, resentment, cynicism, and pride

◀ *You can choose to be happy.*

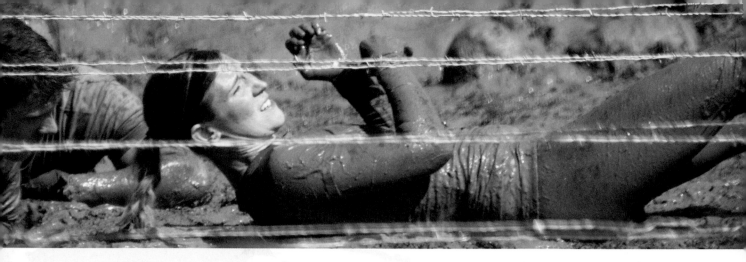

▲ *Commitment has very little to do with feelings.*

- Habits, including sleeping late, watching too much TV, and wasting time

- Addictions: drugs, alcohol, porn, or gambling

Overcoming Obstacles

Conquering one *big* obstacle (external or internal) tends to have a ripple effect in other areas. Just as there are internal and external obstacles, there are internal and external benefits to overcoming obstacles. While the external gains of overcoming an external obstacle may be obvious (the goal on the other side of the obstacle), the internal benefits may be even more valuable. You may gain confidence, character, and wisdom. You may break through fear or eliminate a bad habit. Similarly, when you overcome one of your big *internal* obstacles, you will likely be much better equipped to handle the external.

Here are seven steps to overcoming obstacles:

1. Make a list of the obstacles you currently face.

2. Label them as internal or external.

3. Rate each as small, medium, or BIG.

4. Pick a BIG, external obstacle.

5. What is on the other side of this obstacle? Get very clear on the value of overcoming this obstacle. What would become possible for you?

6. Now look at your internal obstacles. Which of these, if overcome, would enable you to conquer your external obstacle?

7. Get to work on the internal obstacle.

Do it anyway. Pay attention. Approach your internal obstacles with the same fervor and tenacity that you apply to your obstacle challenges. This is the recipe for finding motivation, or what I like to call Muddervation.

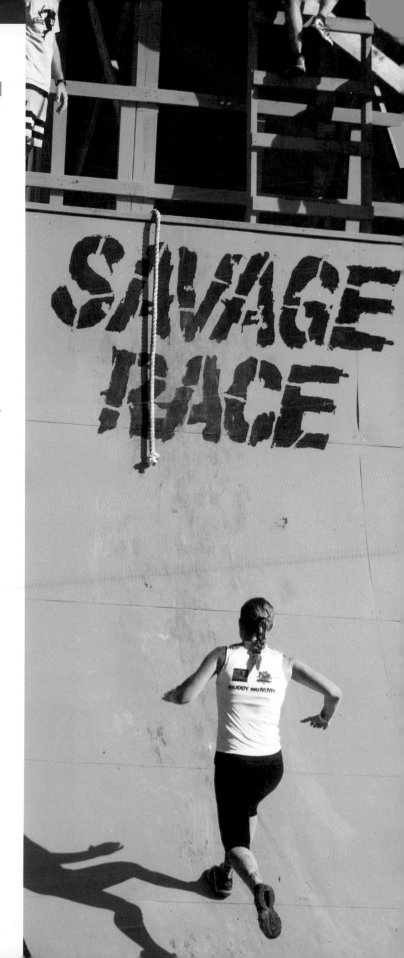

DOWN AND DIRTY TAKEAWAYS

- **Make a commitment.** When you feel like skipping a workout or a run, do it anyway. Watch how great you feel afterward.
- **Increase your awareness and attention.** Ask the right questions. Celebrate your wins. What you put your attention to, you get more of.
- **Overcome obstacles big and small.** Review the seven steps to overcoming obstacles. For further reading, check out Doug's book *The Ripple Effect*.

Doug Grady is an entrepreneur, musician, and author of The Ripple Effect. *He is president of High Achievers, helping people embrace a lifestyle of achievement. His companies, writings, trainings, and music are designed with one purpose: to help people reach their God–given potential. Doug also wrote "The (Unofficial) Tough Mudder Song." Visit www.highachieversnetwork.com for more information.*

▶ *Many times these obstacles are a metaphor for things in your life.*

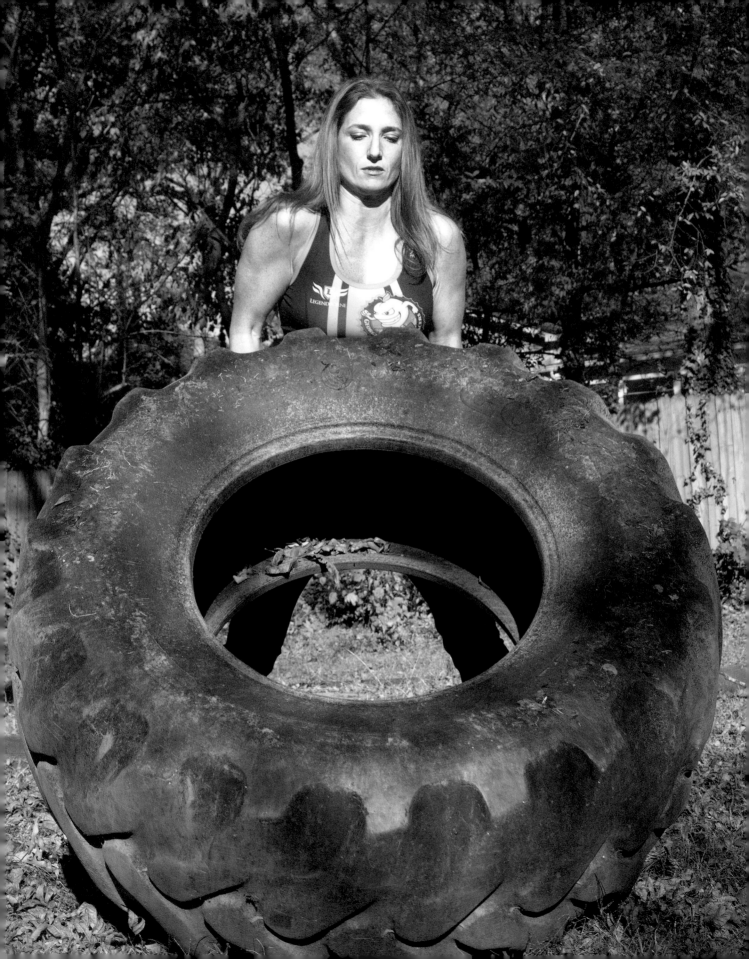

14 CREATING A BACKYARD OBSTACLE COURSE

One of the greatest things about training for obstacle course races is that you don't need to go anywhere or belong to a gym or CrossFit box.

In this chapter, I will tell you how you can create fun, challenging workouts that will allow you to work all kinds of muscles. You can prepare obstacle course races without leaving the comfort of your backyard or neighborhood. I'll give you step-by-step instructions to build sandbags, car tires, tractor tires, and walls. For each project, the costs are approximate and may vary.

Sandbags

Let's start with the least expensive and easiest to obtain and put together. You can buy the materials you'll need from any nearby hardware store.

MATERIALS NEEDED

- 50 pounds (22.7 kg) sand
- 1 box "Demo" Bags (or garbage bags you already own; use three per sandbag)
- Large roll duct tape

1. Open the demo bags, and then pour the sand into the bag or bags. (If you're using garbage bags, you need to layer three bags together to have enough strength so the sandbag doesn't fall apart.) I suggest starting with 20 to 25 pounds (9.1 to 11.3 kg) of sand.

2. Mold the sandbag with your hand to the desired shape. The most common shapes people make are the "brick" or the "burrito." You can personalize your sandbag with marker or colored duct tape.

◄ A giant tire is an awesome OCR training tool; they can be found more easily than you think.

3. Wrap the bag(s) with the duct tape over and over again. You want to pick it up and flip it a few times as you are making it to make sure no sand is loose or falling out. If you have done it correctly, you will not need to reapply tape for a few months, depending on use.

4. Decorate your sandbag, if you wish. A woman in our local OCR group used orange tape to make her sandbag, and she calls it her "Baby Cheeto." Another racer used red tape, and when it turned out to weigh 23 pounds (10.4 kg), she named it "MJ" after Michael Jordan.

If making your own sandbags doesn't sound like fun to you, you can buy sand "bells," which were made popular by Spartan Race. They come empty or filled with sand, and prices vary.

SANDBAG WORKOUT

Now that you've made (or bought) sandbags or bells, the first exercise you can do is simply bring it with you and carry it for all or part of your run. For example, many people in our local OCR group will bring a sandbag along to our favorite local mountain. We will do a 2- to 3-mile (3.2- to 4.8-km) trail run at or near the mountain without the sandbags, then walk up and down the mountain again with the sandbag (gaining about 1,000 feet [300 m]

of elevation). Some people in the group repeat this multiple times, but for others, once in a morning is a perfect workout. You can also create a loop in your neighborhood where, at the end of the loop, you carry the sandbag for a few hundred yards of that loop.

There are a myriad of things to do with sandbags as you get going. You can do lunges, deep knee bends, and presses over your head all while holding your sandbag.

Car Tire

The next item for the homemade obstacle course is the tire. Any standard car tire will do. You can go to a tire store or junkyard, and they might even give them to you for free. Once you start looking for tires, you may notice that people leave them next to dumpsters or by the side of the road.

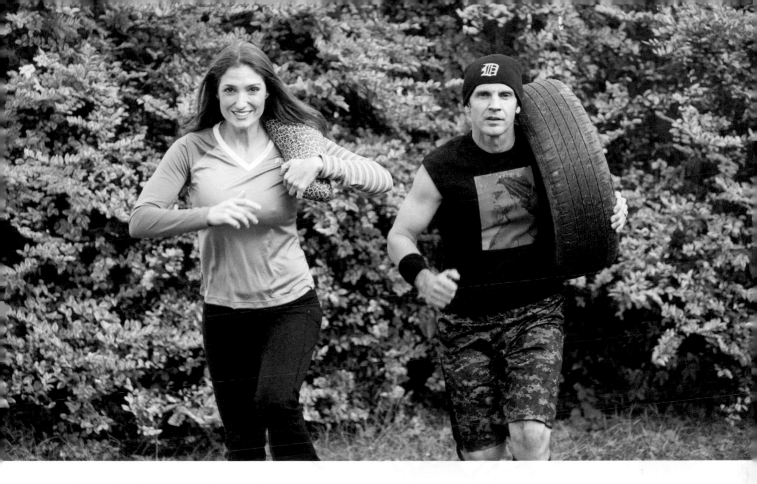

▲ *Inviting friends makes training more fun.*

MATERIALS NEEDED

- Car tire

- Drill (optional)

- Dish towel (optional)

- Duct tape (optional)

1. You can simply grab a tire and go. But some people drill holes in the side of the tire so that water does not collect during rain. (Be sure to drill into the side and not the tread itself. Drilling into the tread will tear up your drill bit).

2. When carrying the tire for long periods, it can tend to dig into the shoulder, so you can add duct tape or a dishtowel for comfort.

3. If you like accessorizing, you can add different kinds and colors of tape for some added flare.

CAR TIRE WORKOUT

The tire is very similar to the sandbag in that you can carry it for any part of your run or workout. If you have the space in your garage or backyard to store several tires, you can do several other activities as well. You can arrange them "football practice" style and run through them, alternating feet. You can also stack them and do box jumps.

This short video from Joel "Dirty" Getty of Inside Obstacle News shows you several ways to work out with the tire: http://tinyurl.com/downanddirtytire.

Tractor Tire
MATERIALS NEEDED

- Tractor tire: (Like their smaller brothers, these tires can also be obtained for free just by asking. Do an Internet search, or ask your local tire dealer where you can get large "farm vehicle" tires or "tractor" tires. These range in weight from 75 to 350 pounds (34 to 160 kg).

TRACTOR TIRE WORKOUT

The exercise that you can do that you will most likely see in an actual obstacle race is the tire flip. Lay the tire on its side, and then flip it a few times forward and back. This will mimic what you'll see at a Spartan Race. I have seen this obstacle at many other races as well.

Flip the tire three times forward and three times backward. Add reps as you get stronger.

The Obstacle Wall

This is something that you need to plan a few hours for. I also recommend getting an obstacle buddy or two to help because first, it will make the job easier and second, OCR peeps do it together.

For this specific wall, we asked OCR fanatic Jonathan Stanizzi to put together his directions.

MATERIALS NEEDED

- Seven boards 2" × 4" × 8'4" (38 mm × 89 mm × 2.5 m)

- Six boards 2" × 6" × 12'6" (cut to 6') (38 mm × 140 mm × 3.81 m) (cut to 1.8 m)

▶ *Add a wall to your backyard, and you have an instant obstacle course!*

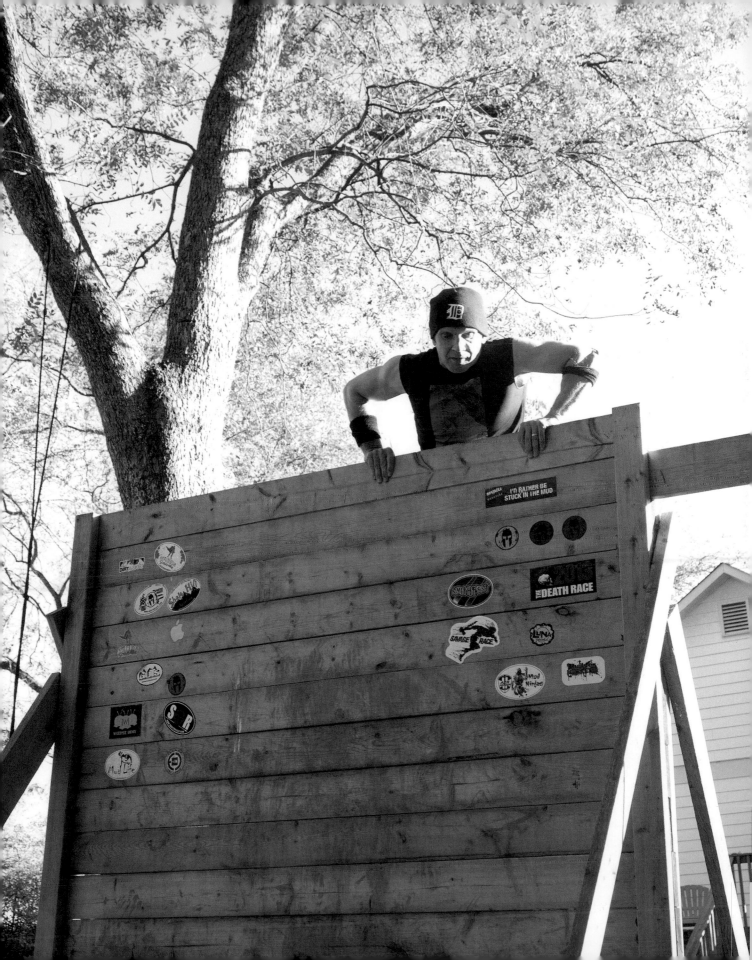

- Two boards 2" × 4" × 10' 4" (38 mm × 89 mm × 3.1 m)

- Two boards 4" × 4" × 8' 4" (89 mm × 89 mm × 2.5 m)

- 2 pounds #8 × 3" (76.2) coarse polymer-coated steel bugle head Phillips exterior screws

- Four 6" (50.8 mm) zinc-plated corner braces

- Six ³/₈" (9.5 mm) × 3-½" (88.9 mm) zinc lag screws

TOOLS NEEDED

- Screw gun

- ¼" (6.35 mm) drill bit

- Skill saw

- Socket wrench

- Miter saw

Note: I bought six 2" × 6" × 12' 6" (38 mm × 140 mm × 3.81 m) boards and had the store cut them into twelve 6' (1.8 m) lengths. This will save you the time of having to do it at home.

1. Lay out two of the 2" × 4" × 8's on the ground approximately 6 feet (1.8 m) apart, and begin to lay the 2" × 6" × 6' boards over the top, width-wise. Don't worry about the 2" × 4"s on the bottom being perfectly lined up because this is simply to hold the 2" × 6"s off of the ground, and you will adjust and screw them in later.

2. Lay out six of the 2" × 6"s, beginning approximately 30 inches (762 mm) from the bottom and then one 2" × 4" × 10', followed by the remaining six 2" × 6"s. At the very top, add the second of the 2" × 4" × 10's. (Note: The two 10' (3 m) boards go in an opposite direction, creating what will be a muscle up/dip bar in the middle and a pull-up bar at the top.)

3. Once all of your boards are in place, lay out two more of the 2" × 4" × 8' boards over the top, sandwiching the 2" × 6"s in between. Line up each of these 2" × 4"s with the edge of the 2" × 6"s. Before you begin screwing, it is essential that you measure from the bottom of the 2" × 4"s to the lowest 2" × 6" on either side to ensure that the board is equidistant from the bottom. Also, make sure that the boards are even with the top of the 2" × 4"s. (Note: We left about a 2" (50.8 mm) gap

▶ *Race your friends!*

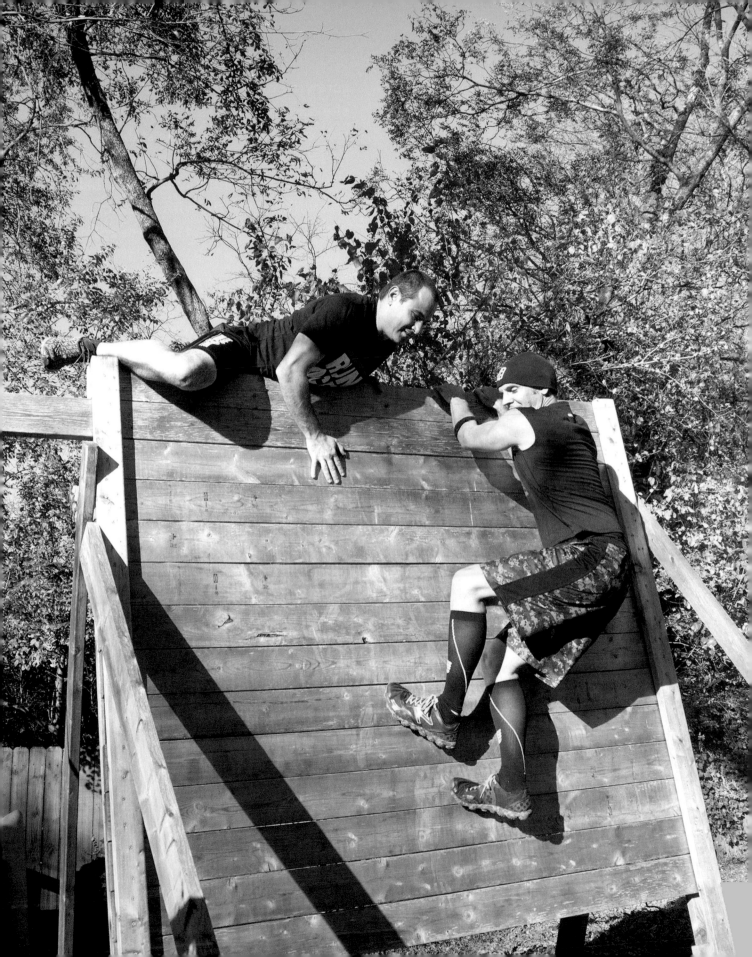

from the top of our wall to the top of the 2" × 4"s.)

Once you have the 2" × 6"s level, and you have the 2" × 4"s in place, you can start to screw the boards together. Remember to begin at the bottom and work your way up the wall. Screw in the boards in a zigzag pattern up the wall. (Note: We did not screw in the muscle-up bar. It can be removed to allow kids a handhold.) Make sure to screw in the 2" × 6" just above the muscle-up bar. This will ensure that the muscle-up bar does not move. The remaining five boards at the top will not be screwed in so that you can slide them in and out to adjust the height of your wall.

Screw in the 2" × 4" × 10' (pull-up bar) at the top. It is important to attach this board to ensure stability when doing pull-ups. (Note: When you lower the wall by removing the top 2" × 6"s, the 2" × 4" × 10' will remain in place.)

The following step may take a few extra hands. Hold tight to either side of the 2" × 4" × 8's, and flip the wall over. Adjust and begin screwing in 2" × 4"s as you did on the other side. When

screwing these in, zigzag in the opposite direction as was done on the other side of the wall to add the stability.

There will be a gap between the two 2" × 4"s at the bottom of the wall that you will want to fill with an extra piece of 2" × 4". Measure the distance from the bottom of the lowest 2" × 6" to the bottom of the 2" × 4"s. Cut two pieces of wood the same length, and slide them into place and secure them.

Once all the 2" × 4"s and 2" × 6"s are secured together, you can stand the wall upright onto the 4" × 4" × 8's. Center the wall on the 4" × 4"s. Put the corner braces in place on either side of the wall and drill pilot holes. Secure all four corner braces with the lag screws, using a socket wrench.

Add the A frame supports on either side of the wall. Cut four 2" × 4"s at an angle with the miter saw so they meet approximately 5 feet (1.5 m) off the ground, and attach them to the upright 2" × 4"s, then secure them to the 4" × 4"s. This will add strength and stability. Connect two horizontal pieces at a height that is just under the muscle-up bar.

Add a piece of wood directly under the pull-up bar. Make sure you do not screw into the top 2" × 6" if you want the option of lowering your wall.

WALL WORKOUT

The obstacle wall is one of the greatest investments you can make if you want to train seriously for OCR. If all you did was use it to go up and over several times a day, you would be a better obstacle course racer. However, there is much more. The pull-up bar and muscle-up bar allow you to work various upper body muscles. The gap at the bottom allows you to practice crawling or rolling under, which mimics barbed wire crawls or the Over-Under-Through obstacle that you see at most obstacle races.

You can also personalize your obstacle wall with paint or stickers. It's a great conversation starter; your neighbors will wonder what is going on in your backyard. What a way to enroll them in their first obstacle course race. I guarantee just having the wall will make you the envy of your OCR friends.

Spear Practice

This project was submitted by obstacle course racer LeEarl Rugland.

MATERIALS NEEDED

- Rake handle
- 12" (30.5 cm) spike
- 4 to 8 hay bales
- Metal saw
- Drill
- $3/8$" (1 cm) wood spade bit
- Hammer

I like to use a 52" (132 cm) handle. It's common to find, and the hole in the end is just slightly smaller than my $3/8$" (1 cm) wood bit. Also the nail fits nice and tight without any glue. Find a handle that has the hole drilled in the center. This will help keep the wood tip from breaking while practicing. Remember to wear eye and hand protection when using hand and power tools.

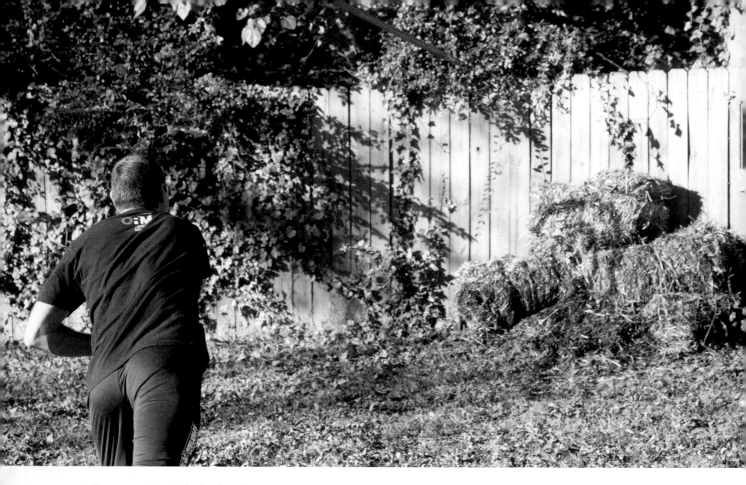

▲ *Spear practice in the backyard . . .*

1. Use your metal saw and cut the head off the nail. This will be the end you pound into your handle so the cut does not need to be perfect.

2. Drill the hole deeper in the rake handle. This will create a deeper hole for the nail where the wood is thicker in the handle. Make sure you keep your hole straight because this will create a nice straight spear point.

3. Using the hammer, tap the nail into the handle. Place the cut end into the handle first and tap the tip of the nail until you hit the bottom of the hole. Make sure the nail is all the way seated into the handle. You should have about 6" (15 cm) of nail showing out the end of your handle.

SPEAR WORKOUT

Spartan Race doesn't reveal exact dimensions for their obstacles. Conventional wisdom states the distance for the spear throw is somewhere between 20 and 30 feet (6.1 and 9.1 m).

1. Stand 25 feet (7.6 m) from your hay bales and start throwing.

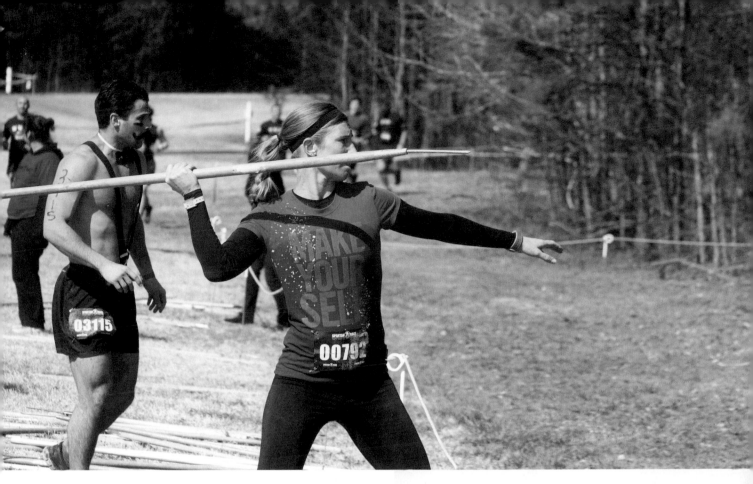

▲ . . . *helps you nail it on race day.*

2. Vary your style of throwing. There is overhand "javelin" style. There is underhand "pool cue" style. There is also the "tomahawk" end-over-end style. It's best to practice various throws to find out what works best for you.

You can just throw that puppy all day and increase your accuracy, or you can play some fun games. The most popular is a version of HORSE that is typically played with a basketball. You and your friend line up and attempt to throw the spear into the hay bales from various spots in the yard. When you make it,

your friend has to make the same shot. If he/she misses, they get the first letter in HORSE , the "H." You keep going until someone spells HORSE. You could change HORSE to PIG to shorten the game. You can get very crafty if you put your mind to it. You can call "left-handed," "eyes closed," or choose various spots on the hay bales to aim for, such as "top left" or "bottom quadrant."

There is a saying that it takes 10,000 efforts to master something. So get started!

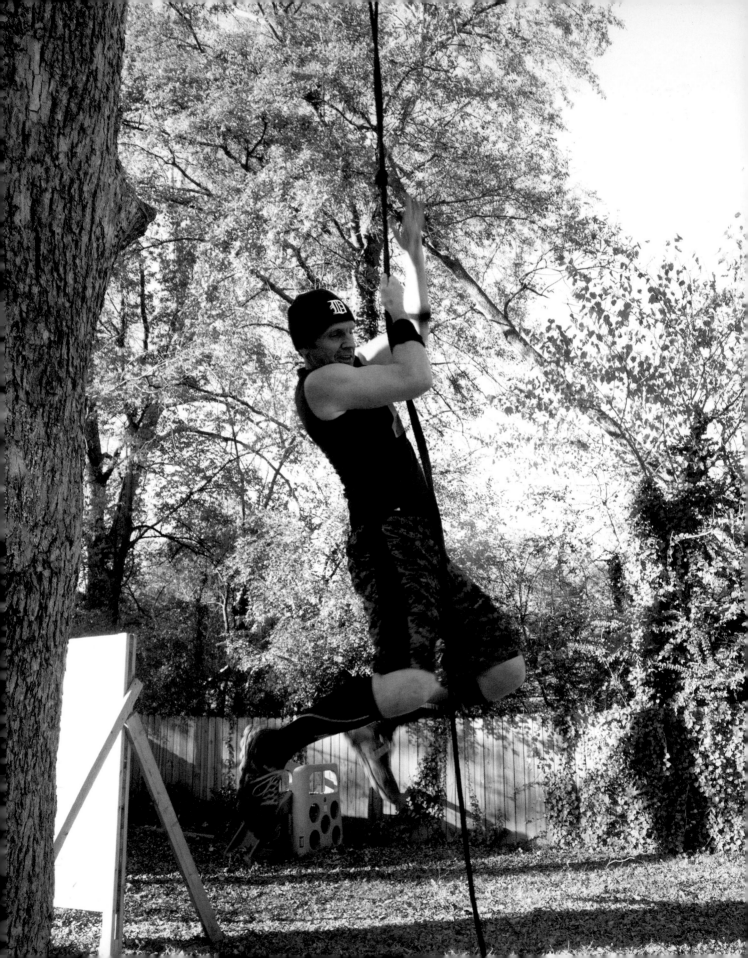

Creating Your Backyard Course

Being able to work out and practice various aspects of obstacle course racing is lots of fun on its own. However, you can take it up another notch by staging your own mini obstacle race with all of your OCR friends.

Here is a sample obstacle course that I made in my backyard and neighborhood. I invited several friends over for a barbecue/obstacle play day. We had a lot of fun competing with each other for the best overall times. You can adjust your course, based on your own yard, neighborhood, and homemade obstacles.

- Start with your hand touching the back fence.
- Run under the 10-foot (3-m) wall.
- Flip the tractor tire three times forward and three times back.
- Run to the front yard.
- Pick up the sandbag, run down the street to a mailbox a few houses down and back.
- Drop the sandbag, pick up the tire.

- Run with the tire all the way to the nearby children's playground 0.25 miles (0.4 km) away.
- When you get to the playground, do the monkey bars.
- Do three hill repeats before exiting the playground.
- Run back to the house.
- Enter the backyard, drop the tire, jump the fire pit.
- Throw the spear; get a burpee penalty for missing.
- Climb the 10-foot (3-m) wall and run through the finish line.

◄ *Tree plus rope equals rope climb practice.*

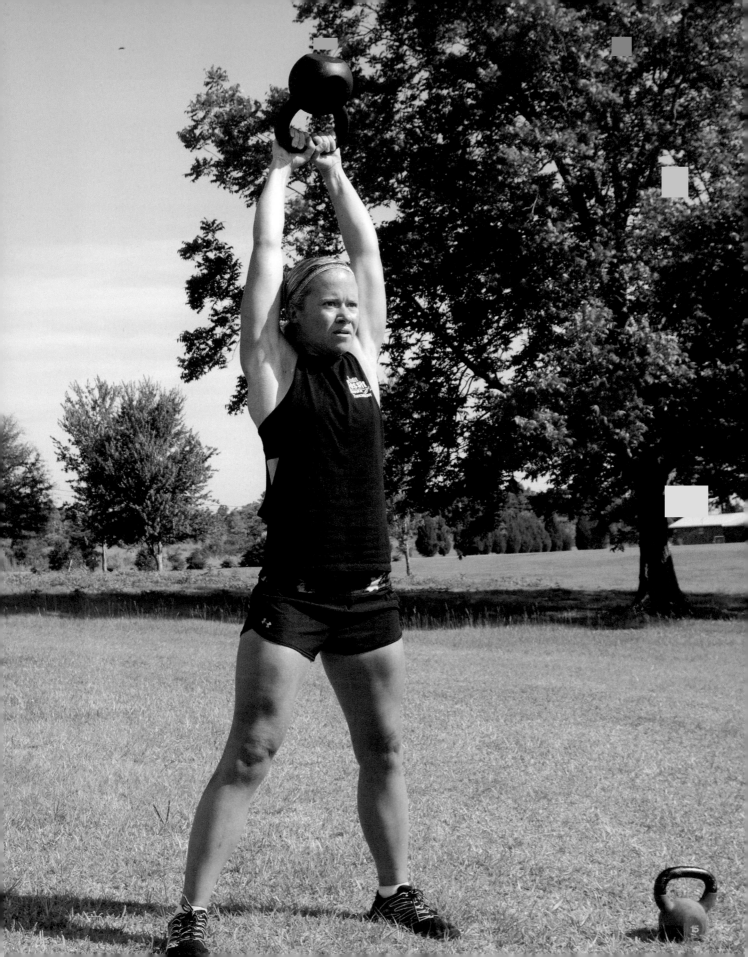

15 ADDING CROSSFIT TRAINING

☙ Featuring CrossFit box owner Janice Marie Ferguson

I'm dedicating an entire chapter to CrossFit because I have heard from so many people in OCR who have received benefits and excelled at OCR after training at a CrossFit box (a.k.a. gym). Like plyometrics, which we discussed in an earlier chapter, CrossFit can benefit your overall fitness as it applies to conquering obstacles.

Janice Marie Ferguson tried CrossFit and, in a very short time, realized amazing benefits as it relates to obstacle course racing. I asked her to contribute this chapter to give you some background on CrossFit and the benefits to OCR.

❧ ❧ ❧

Before we begin, we have to get a few things straight about CrossFit. You're probably reading this chapter with one of three preconceived notions:

1. You love CrossFit and have already witnessed the amazing level of fitness attained through practicing it.

2. You've seen others getting super fit, strong, and fast, and you want to know more about CrossFit.

3. You hate CrossFit, or perhaps you don't see any value in it, for various reasons.

I hope anyone who falls into the third category will read this with an open mind and walk away with a more enlightened perspective. I am contributing this chapter in this book because I believe that CrossFit can be one of many tools that

◀ *Kettlebell swings are a staple of many CrossFit workouts.*

anyone uses to improve their obstacle course racing ability.

I've heard many people describe CrossFit as a cult, passing fad, or even dangerous. I've also heard many stories about how CrossFit literally saved peoples' lives, made them better people inside and out, gave them the freedom to pursue just about any physical and mental challenge, and helped them find a greater purpose in life. I wouldn't be doing you a service if I didn't reveal my bias here. I fall into the latter category, if you haven't noticed already. I also own a CrossFit affiliate. I promise to be as objective as possible while I help you understand CrossFit as it relates to OCR training.

A History of CrossFit

CrossFit was founded by Greg Glassman, a gymnast, in 2000. Glassman defined fitness as three things.

ACHIEVING PROFICIENCY IN TEN GENERAL PHYSICAL SKILLS:

1. Cardio-respiratory endurance
2. Stamina
3. Strength
4. Flexibility
5. Power
6. Speed
7. Coordination
8. Agility
9. Balance
10. Accuracy

PERFORMING WELL AT ANY AND ALL TASKS. This includes competency in doing things you are unfamiliar with. Back flips? Spear throwing? Swinging from rope to rope? Running up endless mountain ski slopes? In essence, a truly fit person would be able to adapt to any of those tasks well.

PROFICIENCY IN THE THREE METABOLIC ENERGY PATHWAYS:

1. Phosphagen, which is high-powered activity lasting less than 10 seconds
2. Glycogen, which is moderate-powered activity lasting up to several minutes
3. Oxidative, which is low-powered activity lasting more than several minutes

The purpose of this three-pronged approach to defining fitness is to create an overall fit individual who has very few weaknesses and no specialty—a jack-of-all-trades, if you will. Glassman has stated many times, "Our specialty is not specializing."

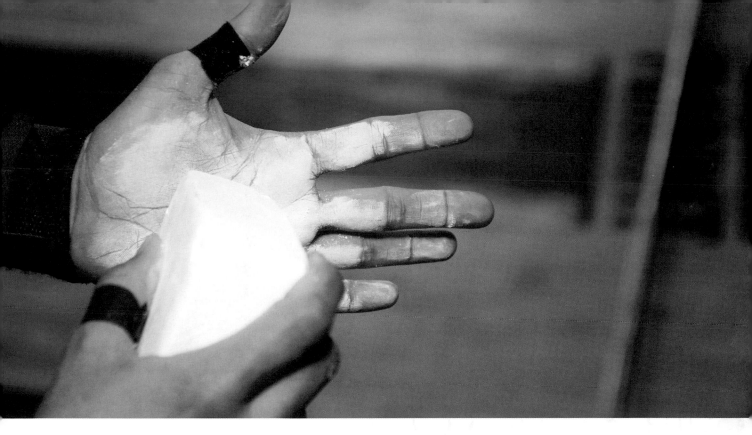

▲ *An athlete chalks up before a CrossFit workout.*

With that definition of fitness, Glassman then defined CrossFit as three things in concert: functional movement, performed at high intensity, across broad time and modal domains. In other words, CrossFitters strive to be ready for anything life could throw their way. To get that readiness, we're consistently working to improve upon the physical skills. We're constantly challenging our ability to master those skills with a variety of tasks, and we're testing our ability to complete those tasks across different levels of intensity/load and time domains.

CrossFit Basics

As a CrossFit affiliate owner, I often get asked, "What is CrossFit? Is that Insanity or P90X?" It's not like any of those programs. Although CrossFit is definitely high-intensity interval training, like many other forms of fitness, P90X, Insanity, etc., that is not the only thing we do in CrossFit.

CrossFitters want to master everything—from running, to gymnastics, to Olympic weightlifting. We want to know all the tips and tricks to becoming a better rower, swimmer, and power lifter. Learning all the finer points of

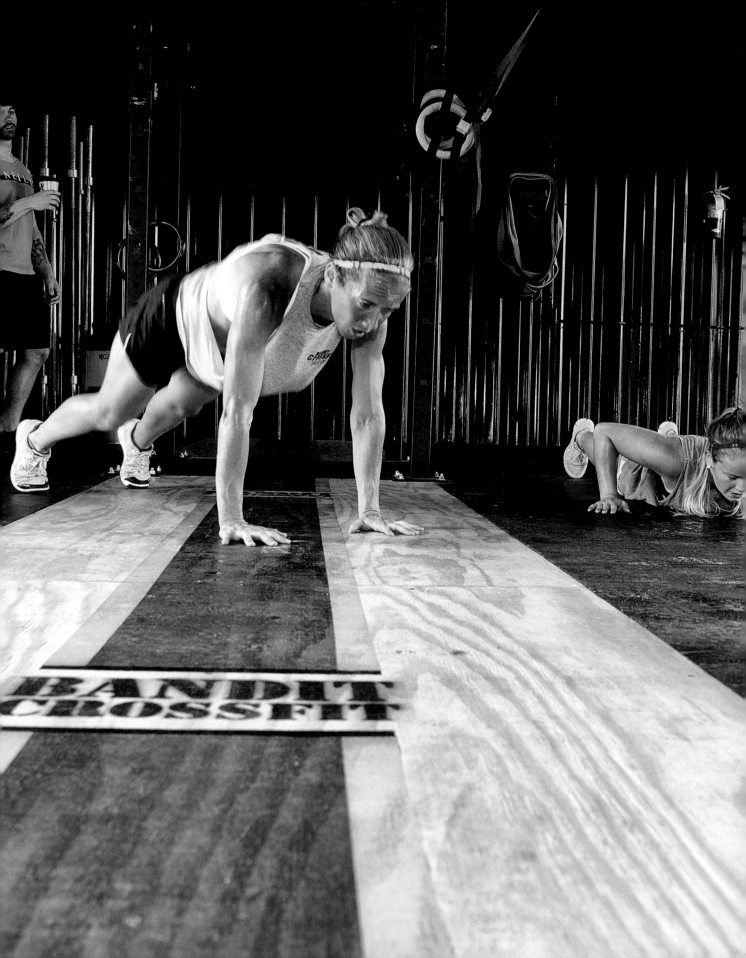

kettle bell swinging and double unders are a must on our list of things to do. We lift weights. We pick stuff up and put it down—not just barbells with bumper plates, but sandbags, and medicine balls, and atlas stones.

CrossFit offers multiple specialty certifications and seminars for people who want to learn more about particular disciplines. Many CrossFit affiliates even offer classes tailored to those specialties, such as CrossFit Endurance.

CrossFitters fancy themselves as scientists or mad chemists in the arena of improving sports performance. CrossFit is data- and results-based. We want to see measurable results in our progress. We also want to dissect what professional athletes have been doing for strength and conditioning and see how it can be improved upon. Resources that were once only available to the top athletes in the country and world on the topics of training, sleep, recovery, performance, and nutrition are now tested and are open-source discussions for thousands of everyday people like you and me. CrossFit means access to what the pros do. This means increased performance for the masses.

CrossFit focuses on efficient movement and proper technique. Efficient movement is one of the hallmarks of CrossFit. We also know that technique must come before load or intensity. This concentration on technique and movement efficiency has great application and transfer for obstacle racing success, or any other sports performance goal. Moving efficiently saves energy. Saving energy saves time. In sports and competitive performance, where every second counts, the most efficient athletes come out on top time and time again.

CrossFit founder Glassman stated many times that the greatest adaptation in CrossFit is not what happens to the physical body, but what happens to a person between the ears—their mentality. I know this to be true. This is the part that makes CrossFit so addictive. Every day in my CrossFit routine, I do something, even small things, better than I could do the last time. I may run a little faster. Or I do one more pull-up. Or I put more weight on my bar. Making gains and progress is very satisfying. It also teaches you the value of hard work in attaining your goals. Over time, you begin to change

◄ *Find a CrossFit box (aka gym) in your town that's the right fit for you.*

your mindset. Things that used to seem impossible become possible.

Another aspect of CrossFit is the competitive nature. Every day, you go to the gym, you are "racing" someone. You want to lift more weight, run or row faster, or do more pull-ups. Over the course of nearly four years, CrossFit has prepared me mentally and physically to take on any challenge or put myself to the test in just about any way imaginable. Obstacle racing is just one of those tests.

CrossFit training, according to Glassman's definition of fitness, has direct application to obstacle racing. It cannot be argued that the ten general physical skills are all necessities for the sport of obstacle racing. It's obvious that some of those skills are weighted more heavily than others, especially for those who are hoping to stay in the ranks of the elite obstacle racers. However, if you are someone who merely wants to do these races for the sake of completion, you may be able to get away with less focus on specific training, and more general physical preparedness, also known as GPP in CrossFit. In fact, I completed my very first Spartan Race, in 2012, in the midst of a strength cycle—heavy dead lifts, squats, and very short conditioning workouts. It wasn't just any Spartan Race. It was the Pennsylvania Sprint, which is a tough

course located on a ski resort. The climbing was endless, but I was well prepared to complete the race, and I did so with no burpee penalties. I attribute that to CrossFit.

Using CrossFit for OCR

Now that you know what CrossFit is, and how it can benefit your training, it's time to implement it. To maximize the benefits of CrossFit, there are a few things to consider.

SET SOME GOALS. Do you dream of ranking among the elite obstacle racers? Or are you happy just completing the races and improving every time?

If you have dreams of toeing the start line with today's top racers, you'll certainly need to have a more purposeful or specialized type of training. A great program tailored for endurance athletes with the benefits of CrossFit is known as CrossFit Endurance. I highly recommend this program, or at the very least taking components from it and adding them to your training. While CrossFit can certainly be used as one of many tools, you will definitely need to spend some time in sport-specific training, especially with the caliber of athletes who are racing and will be racing in the future.

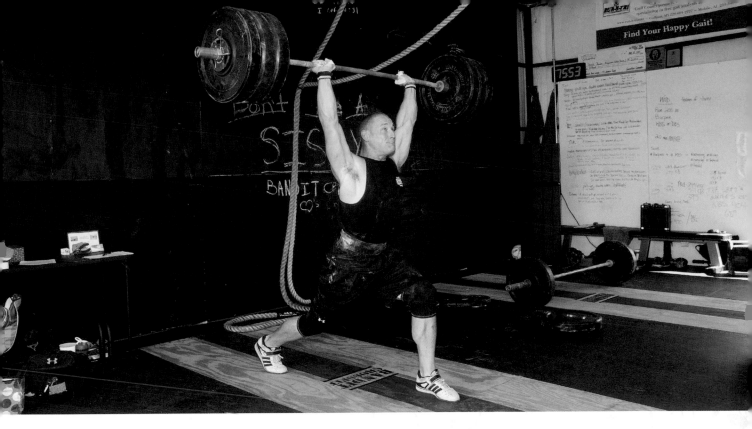

▲ *Improving strength through weightlifting is not required for OCR, but it may help.*

If you're happy running the race for the experience with friends, a generalized CrossFit program designed to maximize your GPP, mixed with some longer efforts for practicing race-day nutrition, electrolyte replacement, and hydration could very well be your ticket to success.

CHOOSE YOUR TYPE OF TRAINING: INDEPENDENT OR SOCIAL. If you're an independent, do-it-yourself type of person, you might want to try CrossFit on your own and integrate it into your own exercise routine. The CrossFit and CrossFit Endurance websites are great places to start. Also, the online *CrossFit Journal* has thousands of articles and resources, and you can connect with other CrossFitters on their online message board. Brian MacKenzie, of CrossFit Endurance, has a host of videos and even a book, *Power, Speed, Endurance: A Skill-Based Approach to Endurance Training*, that would be a great place to start for someone looking to implement CrossFit into their obstacle course race training routine. You don't need to go to a gym to do CrossFit. You can work out in your very own garage or at a local park. A jump rope, sandbag, and kettle bell can take you a long way.

On the other hand, if you crave a social experience or need extra motivation or instruction, you might want to join a CrossFit gym. If you choose this route, it's paramount that you do your homework and shop around, so you can find the best fit for you. Take a look at the workouts for a couple of weeks at the gyms in your area. Most CrossFit affiliates post their workouts daily for the members and public to see. What kind of work are they doing? Look at the pictures on their websites and social media channels. What type of events do their members frequent? Ask to try the gym out for a few days to see if you fit in, and if you are receiving the kind of attention and instruction you need from the coaching staff.

All CrossFit gyms are different. That is the beauty of CrossFit. Each affiliate owner has the freedom to express fitness in his or her own way. Find the gym that fits you and your goals. No matter which gym you choose, though, you should expect high-quality instruction and programming no matter what the focus: endurance, weightlifting, gymnastics, etc.

DOWN AND DIRTY TAKEAWAYS

- **Mix it up.** CrossFit's specialty is *not* specializing.
- **Focus on technique.** Technique must come before load or intensity. Learn to move correctly so you minimize injury risk and perform at your best.
- **Maximize your genetics.** Believe it or not, we are not all born the same. However, CrossFit can help you maximize what nature gave you.
- **Set goals.** Figuring out your goals can help you decide which training regimen will best suit you.
- **Shop around.** Each CrossFit gym is different. Explore some different places. Most of them offer a free one-day trial. Find out what works for you.

Janice Marie Ferguson, head coach and owner of Bandit CrossFit, is a wife and mother with a passion for obstacle course racing and CrossFit. She is a 2012 South Central CrossFit Games Regional Individual Qualifier and a two-time Spartan Race podium finisher. She also races for Team Obstacle Racing Media, which finished as the first-place team in four straight Superhero Scramble races in 2013. Learn more on her website at www.janicemarieferguson.blogspot.com

CROSSFIT RESOURCES

CrossFit Theory and General Information Websites

CrossFit: www.crossfit.com

CrossFit Endurance: www.crossfitendurance.com

CrossFit Journal: http://journal.crossfit.com

CrossFit message board: http://board.crossfit.com

Injury, Mobility, and Efficient Movement

Mobility WOD: www.mobilitywod.com

Pose Running: www.posetech.com

Olympic Weightlifting Sites

Catalyst Athletics: www.catalystathletics.com

USA Weightlifting: www.teamusa.org/USA-Weightlifting

CrossFit Gyms and Other Sites I Follow for Workout Ideas:

Outlaw CrossFit: http://outlawcrossfit.com

Gymnastics WOD: http://gymnasticswod.com

Travel WODs/WODs with minimal equipment: http://stayforevercrossfit.com/extras/wods-to-go/

Spartan Race WOD: www.spartanrace.com/wod/

Nutrition

Eat to Perform: http://eattoperform.com

Robb Wolf: http://robbwolf.com

Loren Cordain: http://thepaleodiet.com

The Zone Diet: http://www.zonediet.com

Whole 9: http://whole9life.com

Books

Pose Method of Running, Nicholas Romanov with John Robson

Power, Speed, Endurance: A Skill Based Approach to Endurance Training, Brian MacKenzie

Olympic Lifting: A Complete Guide for Athletes and Coaches, Greg Everett

Becoming a Supple Leopard: The Ultimate Guide to Resolving Pain, Reducing Injury and Improving Athletic Performance, Kelly Starrett

Paleo Diet for Athletes, Loren Cordain, Joe Friel

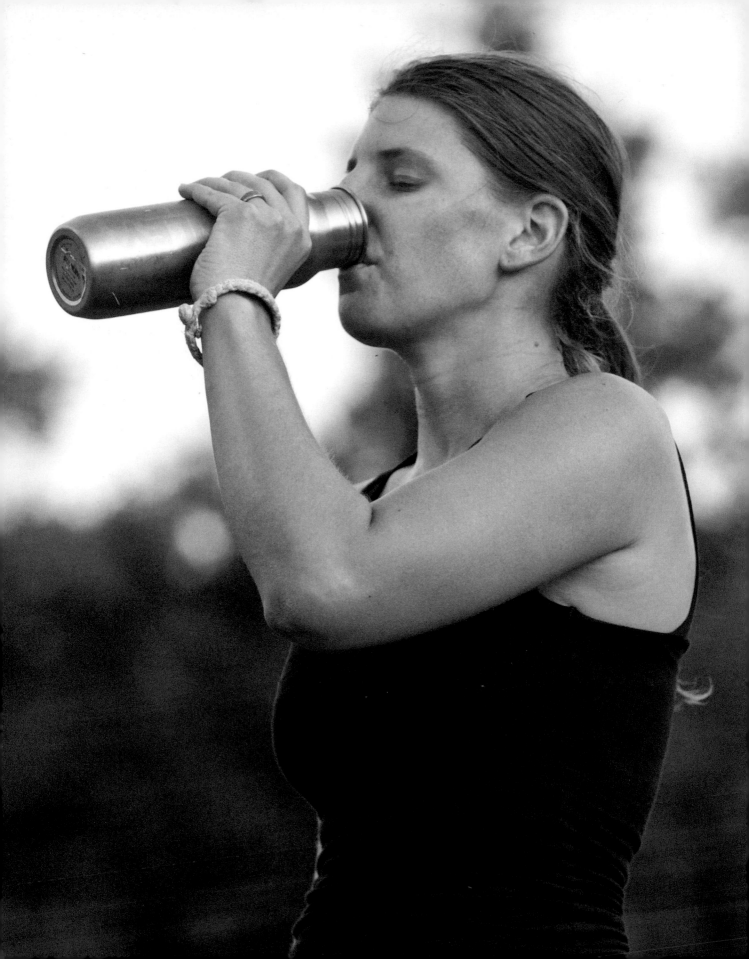

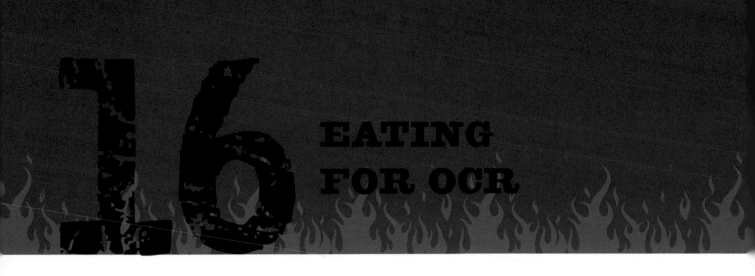

⚑ **Featuring elite Spartan Pro Team racer Alec Blenis and Death Race winner Nele Schulze**

We could fill libraries with all the books and articles written on health and nutrition. To simplify for the purposes of the book, I thought it would be very helpful to include two nutrition paths that are currently popular in the world of OCR. I asked Alec Blenis to write on plant-based eating, and Nele Schulze to contribute her thoughts on the Paleo diet. These are merely suggestions and, as with gear and the various forms of training, your results may vary. I suggest experimenting and finding out what works best for you.

Plant-Based Diets

I first saw Alec Blenis on video, watching his third place Spartan Race finish in March 2012. A few weeks later, he was so far ahead of me in an ultra-marathon that he passed me going back the other direction. I soon reached out to connect with him via social media, and we've since traveled to many races together.

Alec swears by his diet as one of the contributing factors to consistently making the podium in either his age group or overall (at least fifty times as of this writing), in everything from local 5ks to obstacle races to ultras.

⚑ ⚑ ⚑

"You must train really hard," I often hear, as though hard work is the sole determinant of good performance. So common is the ideology that if you want to be a better runner, you just need to run more; if you want to be a better cyclist, you need

◄ *Food choices and hydration are an important part of any training regimen.*

to cycle more; if you want to be stronger, you need to lift more weight. Rightfully so, a genetic component is also typically used to describe performance. The formula goes something like this: good genes + hard work = performance. This thought process comes so naturally to most people, athletes especially, that the most crucial aspect of their training is often neglected entirely.

In simplest terms, exercise is little more than breaking down muscle tissue to stimulate cellular regeneration. Destroying muscle doesn't sound like much fun, but that second part is key: What would exercise be without recovery? Many people assume that exercise automatically results in recovery; the truth is, exercise does not cause recovery. Your body may recover in response to the stress of exercise, but what happens when that response is inhibited? Is it possible to actually increase your body's response to exercise (and other forms of stress)? If so, that means an athlete could actually train less but perform better. Further, by reducing recovery time between workouts, this athlete could effectively train more frequently and with more intensity if recovery is maintained. Clearly, recovery is key for maximum performance.

What is recovery? More sleep? Ice baths? Massage therapy? Protein shakes?

Recovery comes in many forms, but all can be tied directly to nutrition. Food has the power to rebuild muscle tissue (amino acids), reduce stress on a cellular level (antioxidants), provide instant fuel (carbohydrates) and fuel for the long haul (fatty acids), and much more. Good nutrition is critical for any athlete. This brings us to what constitutes good nutrition.

GOOD NUTRITION THROUGH WHOLE FOODS

Everyone is different. Different people have different lifestyles, training habits, and favorite foods. It's important to find what works for you. A good nutrition plan is one that includes quality energy and nutrients to fuel your active lifestyle, and that's not too rigid or restrictive. A good nutrition plan is one that you enjoy and can stick with.

I personally adhere to and recommend a 100 percent whole-food, plant-based diet. (In practice, it's more like 80 percent whole food, 100 percent plant-based, but more on that later.) But what are whole foods and plant-based foods?

WHOLE FOODS: Any fruit, vegetable, nut, seed, grain, legume, or spice that has not been processed in any way that alters its nutritional profile and completeness.

WHOLE FOODS VERSUS INCOMPLETE COUNTERPARTS

Here are some examples of whole foods and incomplete counterparts.

Whole Food	Incomplete Food
Brown rice	White rice
Whole wheat flour	Bleached enriched flour
Coconut water	Cola
Whole milk	Nonfat milk

Other incomplete foods include refined sugar, starches, and oils.

ANIMAL-BASED VERSUS PLANT-BASED FOODS

Here are some examples of animal-based foods and superior plant-based alternatives.

Animal-Based	Plant-Based
Cow milk, goat milk	Almond milk, coconut milk, hemp milk
Whey protein powder	Pea protein, hemp protein, rice protein
Fish oil pills	Flaxseed oil, chia seeds
Butter	Coconut oil
Beef chili	Bean chili

Many whole foods are also animal-based foods, and many incomplete foods are actually plant-based. Take away foods that are incomplete and animal-based, and you'll get a list of whole-food, plant-based nutritional powerhouses:

- **Fibrous vegetables:** beets, bell peppers, carrots, celery, cucumbers, spinach, kale, collard greens, zucchini, squash, and chard
- **Legumes:** black beans, red lentils, black-eyed peas, kidney beans, and green peas
- **Pseudograins:** quinoa, wild rice, buckwheat, and amaranth
- **Grains:** whole oats, brown rice, kamut, barley, and wheat
- **Seeds:** flax, hemp, sesame, sunflower, pumpkin, and chia
- **Nuts:** almonds, cashews, hazelnuts, walnuts, pine nuts, and pecans
- **Fruit:** apples, apricots, bananas, berries, cherries, dates, figs, grapes, melons, papayas, peaches, pears, pineapples, and plums

PLANT-BASED FOODS: A food that does not contain any animal-based substance or ingredient derived from an animal-based substance. All ingredients are plants, parts of plants, or originated from plants.

This is the basis of good nutrition, and the variety is endless. While these foods are the foundation, other foods such as spices, fermented foods, whole-food supplements, sports nutrition products, healthy sweeteners, and desserts can all be part of a healthy, plant-based diet. Powerful, healthy food does not have to be bland and boring. If your food doesn't taste great, you're doing it wrong.

THE WHOLE FOOD, PLANT-BASED PYRAMID

Remember our old friend, the food pyramid? Here's a better one: The foundation is fibrous vegetables—and not just broccoli, cabbage, carrots, and spinach, but also more unusual varieties such as lotus root, daikon, bok choy, spaghetti squash, and sprouts. Vegetables are rich sources of vitamins, minerals, and antioxidants, and they provide the carbohydrates you need to sustain activity (without spiking blood sugar).

The next level of the whole-food, plant-based pyramid is protein. People love to talk protein! We live in a society that advocates low-fat, low-carb diets and foods and emphasizes protein consumption. Critics of vegan diets often point out that plant foods are incomplete proteins; however, the fact is that the entire notion of complete proteins is outdated and inaccurate. Yes, eating a wide variety of foods to get a full spectrum of amino acids is important, but the apparent need to consume all nine essential amino acids at every meal is not based on science. Studies show that as long as we consume the necessary nutrients and amino acids over the course of a day (or even a week), our bodies have no difficulty synthesizing the proteins we need for proper functioning.

"If your food doesn't taste great, you're doing it wrong."

You can still get complete protein—and lots of it—from plant sources: A Whopper from Burger King has 31 grams of protein and packs 670 calories. For the same amount of calories, you can get 45 grams of protein from black beans, 24 grams from quinoa, 24 grams from almond butter, or 50 grams from broccoli!

The next level of the whole-food, plant-based pyramid is fat. Fat often gets a bad rap, but essential fatty acids (EFAs) are important for good health, and the ability to metabolize fat for fuel is critical for endurance performance. But not just any fat. Look for cold-pressed, unrefined oils such as tea seed, coconut, red palm, avocado, olive, hemp, and flax oil. Those are listed in order of heat stability; oils such as tea seed and coconut are great for cooking because they don't degrade under high heat and have a high flash point; hemp and flax oil should never be heated due to their high omega-3 content.

Speaking of omega-3s, many think you can't get enough of them through a plant-based diet: wrong. In fact, the number one known source of omega-3 on the planet is a plant. *Plukenetia volubilis*, more commonly known as the Sacha Inchi seed, has seventeen times the omega-3s by weight as wild-caught salmon. Chia, flax, hemp, and certain vegetables also contain ample amounts.

WHY FOLLOW A PLANT-BASED DIET?

Plenty of evidence, both observational and empirical, suggests this is the best way to eat (not to mention ethical and environmental concerns, but that is another topic entirely). Here are a few notable vegan athletes.

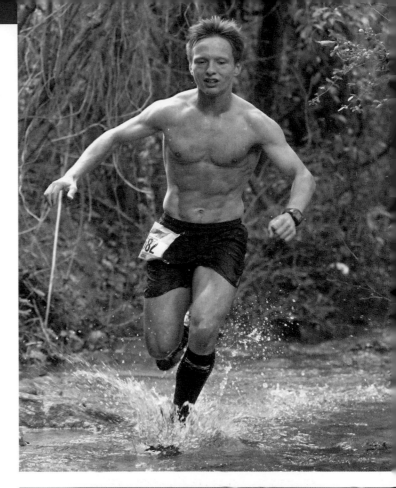

▶ *Alec and Nele both attribute their success in racing to their nutrition plans.*

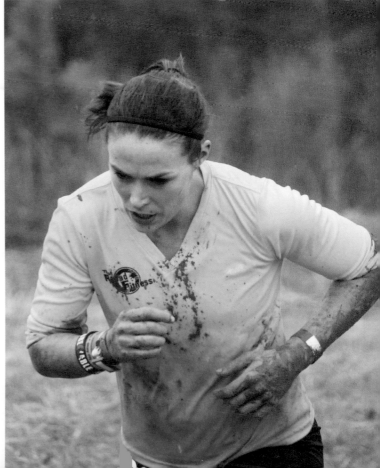

SUN-DRIED TOMATO BROCCOLI SOUP

10 to 16 ounces (283 to 453 g) chopped frozen broccoli thawed

6 ounces (170 g) sun-dried tomatoes, chopped

1 large onion, chopped

3 cloves garlic, peeled and chopped

3 cups (710 mL) chicken broth

Oil of choice for cooking

Salt and pepper to taste

Heat oil of choice in a large saucepan. Sauté the onions and garlic over medium heat until tender, about 8 to 10 minutes. Stir continually so you don't burn the garlic.

Add in broccoli, sun-dried tomatoes, and chicken broth; bring to a boil. Reduce heat, cover, and simmer for 15 minutes or until the vegetables are tender.

Blend in an immersion or regular blender until smooth. Return to the sauce pan on a low heat and season with salt and pepper; serve warm.

Makes 6 servings

Courtesy of www.civilizedcavemancooking.com

RICH ROLL: Top finisher at the Ultraman World Championships (6.2-mile [10-km] swim, 261.1-mile [420.2-km] cross country bike ride, 52.4-mile [84.3-km] run), multi-time finisher of lifestyle for his transformation from overweight and out-of-shape to one of the fittest men on earth.

BRENDAN BRAZIER: Former professional Ironman triathlete and Canadian 50-km (31.1-mi) National Champion and formulator of the award-winning sports nutrition line Vega, he authored *Thrive*, a book advocating a diet much like the one described earlier.

SCOTT JUREK: Ultramarathon runner with multiple wins at Badwater, the Spartathlon, and Western States 100, Jurek also set the American record in the 24-hour run with 165.7 miles (265 km). He adopted a plant-based diet in 1999 to improve his performance and accelerate his recovery.

ENJOYING A WHOLE-FOOD, PLANT-BASED DIET

"But plants don't taste good," you might be thinking. Bad (real) food hardly exists, but bad cooking is everywhere. Not all your food has to be steamed, boiled, or raw (although raw food is great), and you don't have to give up sweets forever. Experiment with different recipes and cooking methods, and you'll surely find something you enjoy. Here are two of my favorite recipes.

PALEO ENERGY BARS

There are also some really delicious desserts you can make. This is my favorite.

1 cup (80 g) shredded coconut + additional to coat balls
3 cups (680 g) pitted dates
1 tablespoon (7 g) ground cinnamon
1 tablespoon (20 g) maple syrup

In a food processor, process 1 cup (80 g) of the coconut for 5 minutes, until smooth. Add the dates and cinnamon, and process for 2 to 3 minutes. Add the maple syrup, and process for 30 seconds. Roll the mixture into balls and toss with the additional shredded coconut to coat.

Makes 10 to 12 small servings

BURRITOS

One of my favorite things to cook is a burrito. The possibilities are endless: beans, veggies, Mexican spices, or something more unique.

1 onion, chopped
1 tablespoon (14 g) coconut oil
½ cup (64 g) diced bell pepper
½ cup (64 g) diced carrot
½ cup (64 g) diced zucchini
2 cups (342 g) beans (black, pinto, or a combination)
Cumin, coriander, cayenne pepper, black pepper, cilantro, to taste
1 tortilla (sprouted wheat or brown-rice) or a collard leaf

In a medium pan, cook the onion in the oil over medium heat until translucent. Add the pepper, carrot, and zucchini. Add the beans. Add cumin, coriander, cayenne pepper, black pepper, and cilantro to taste. Place the mixture into the center of the tortilla or collard leaf and wrap up.

Makes 1 burrito

Alec Blenis is currently on the Spartan Pro Team and is an engineering student at Georgia Tech University in Atlanta.

The Paleo Diet

Nele Schulze has a very sweet disposition in her day-to-day life as a developmental specialist and researcher. She is also a fierce competitor, which everyone in the OCR world became well aware of when she won the 2013 Winter Death Race. I asked her to put down her thoughts on how the Paleo diet helps her to train for obstacle and endurance racing.

❦ ❦ ❦

I have struggled with gastroenterological problems since my teenage years. I'd get stomach pains, I would constantly feel bloated and tired, and I would develop rashes. In June 2012, I fell in love with OCRs, and I began to train for races, but it did not occur to me to change my diet for quite some time.

Sometime later, I met Beth Jones from the New England Spahtens, and she introduced me to Paleo. I had never heard of this diet or lifestyle before. She'd had a fantastic experience with Paleo, and it had become her lifestyle. Then I began CrossFit as a form of cross training, and I noticed how popular Paleo was in the world of CrossFit. With help from my CrossFit gym, Mountain Strength CrossFit in Winchester, Massachusetts, I began to investigate this diet further and

NUTRITION RESOURSES

Plenty of great resources will teach you how to make your food both healthy and delicious. Here are some good places to start.

Thrive, by Brendan Brazier (Da Capo Press, 2008)

Whole, by Dr. Colin Campbell (BenBella Books, 2013)

Crazy Sexy Diet, by Kris Carr (Globe Pequot, 2011)

No Meat Athlete, by Matt Frazier (Fair Winds Press, 2013)

Forks Over Knives (film, 2011)

give it a try. "What's the worst that could happen?" I thought.

At first, I was overwhelmed when I saw what I could and couldn't eat. The list of foods to cut out was long. It was time to hit the books and learn more about Paleo.

The Paleo diet is based on the diets of the people of the Palaeolithic era, which is a period in history that dates from about 2.6 million years ago to roughly 10,000 years ago when stone tools were first developed. The diet consists of predominantly meat and vegetables, some fruit, and some nuts and seeds. It excludes dairy, grains, legumes, and processed food. Essentially, the Paleo diet is a stricter, more-defined version of clean eating.

Personally, the Paleo diet and lifestyle works well for me; I like having strict can/can't eat lists that are very black and white. It's also simple because there is no calorie counting, something I hate doing.

My first week of being on Paleo was tough. I was shocked by how tired I felt, but I knew why. I had drastically cut down on carbs, and my body was fuelling itself differently, and it takes some adjustment. Training during that week was hard. I lacked the motivation I usually had, and so many times I just wanted to be in bed. I even skipped a workout or two to stay home and curl up on the sofa. I knew this was going to happen, and I knew to stick it out.

> "Paleo is a tool to help you listen to your body in terms of diet and find a healthy balance, including what works for you."

After that first week, I started to feel more energetic. It slowly became easier to get up and go run or go to the gym. Working out after work became a breeze.

As the days went by, I noticed that my body was becoming more defined. I felt like I jiggled less when running, and I

FRIED BANANAS

1 ripe banana (or as many as you want to eat)
Coconut oil (for sautéing)
Ground cinnamon

Slice the banana lengthwise. In a medium pan, sauté the banana in the oil until brown and caramelized. Sprinkle with the cinnamon.

Makes 1 serving

had developed a flat stomach. I had spent so much of my time feeling bloated and weighed down that seeing a flat stomach with the beginning of abs blew me away. I had been intensively working out for months, but felt my physical appearance had changed more in the few weeks I had been on Paleo.

Because I wasn't bloated, I felt faster. My times were starting to decrease. I was averaging a 7- to 7:30-minute mile (1.6 km) when previously my average was more around 8- to 8:30-minute mile. The high amounts of protein I was consuming definitely helped my muscle mass, and my strength increased, although not as much as I thought it would.

As an athlete, I had to modify the Paleo diet to work for me. *The Paleo Diet for Athletes* by Loren Cordain is the book

PALEO COOKIES

½ cup (118 ml) coconut oil

2 large eggs

1 very ripe banana

1 ½ teaspoons vanilla

½ cup (118 ml) + 1 tablespoon (15 g)
    coconut flour

½ teaspoon baking soda

Preheat the oven to 350°F (180°C or gas mark 6). Line a baking sheet with parchment paper.

In a medium bowl, combine the oil, eggs, banana, and vanilla.

In a separate bowl, combine the flour and baking soda. Combine the wet and dry mixtures. Spoon out cookie-size amounts onto the baking sheet. Bake for 10 to 12 minutes.

Makes 15–18 cookies

I would most recommend. The Paleo diet is great, but an athlete who trains 6 days a week and participates in 40- to 60-hour endurance events needs to be able to be more flexible with Paleo. *The Paleo Diet for Athletes* helped me find a good balance in terms of my diet. With help from Reload Fitness (a supplement and nutrition company that specializes in the needs of specific athletes), I was able to find a balance within Paleo that worked for me.

I follow the Paleo diet, but in endurance events I do use GU shots or shot blocks, or whatever easy sources of energy work for me. Also, I take a protein shake within 30 minutes of every workout, whether or not it is a Paleo–approved shake. I also have a pre-workout drink that I consume roughly 15 minutes before a workout.

Paleo is a tool to help you listen to your body in terms of diet and find a healthy balance, including what works for you. I think it can be very individualized; for example, some people can tolerate dairy (I, unfortunately, am not one of those people) and include dairy in their diet. Paleo gives me the boundaries I need so I don't eat sugary snacks every single day and then wonder why I feel sick or lack motivation to work out. But by stretching some of the boundaries to include foods that I have tried and tested and that improve my athletic performance, it gives me the flexibility when it's needed.

Friends always say they couldn't try the Paleo diet because they love desserts too much. Two simple dessert recipes that I enjoy are included here.

RESOURCES

The Paleo Diet for Athletes, by Loren Cordain: excellent for breaking down the Paleo diet for athletes

The Paleo Solution, by Robb Wolf: the original, a good read for information about the Paleo diet

Michael Symon's Carnivore, by Michael Symon: not the Paleo diet, but it contains good meat recipes that can be Paleo, just double-check the ingredients

Everyday Paleo, by Sarah Fragoso: great simple recipes as well as an overview of the Paleo diet There are also numerous websites such as www.everydayPaleo.com, which have some great recipes

Nele Schulze is an obstacle course racer who has been racing since June 2012. She lives in New England and feels fortunate to have met a lot of other obstacle course racers in the area. She races and trains with the New England Spahtens and Team Reload Fitness.

CAVEMAN CRUNCH

½ cup (73 g) raw sunflower seeds
½ cup (32 g) raw pumpkin seeds
1 cup (100 g) almond meal
1 cup (80 g) shredded unsweetened coconut
2 cups (290 g) almonds, chopped or slivered
2 tablespoons (16 g) unsweetened cacao powder
Cinnamon to taste
½ cup (118 mL) grape seed oil (or any oil of choice, you can try coconut)
½ cup (118 mL) 100% raw organic honey
1 teaspoon vanilla

Preheat oven to 325°F (170°C, or gas mark 3). In a large mixing bowl, combine the first seven ingredients and mix well.

In a separate bowl, combine oil, honey, and vanilla. If needed, microwave on high for 20 to 30 seconds to help it mix better.

Pour wet ingredients over the dry seed and nut mixture, and mix well with a fork to coat. Place on a foil-lined baking sheet and spread thin and evenly. Bake in the oven for 25 minutes.

Remove from the oven and stir to ensure nothing burns; you can put it back in the bowl and then re-spread it on the baking sheet, if needed. Place back in the oven for 5 minutes. Remove and let cool to let it develop crunchiness and improve taste. Serve in a bowl with some almond milk or coconut milk and enjoy.

Makes 10 servings

Courtesy of www.civilizedcavemancooking.com

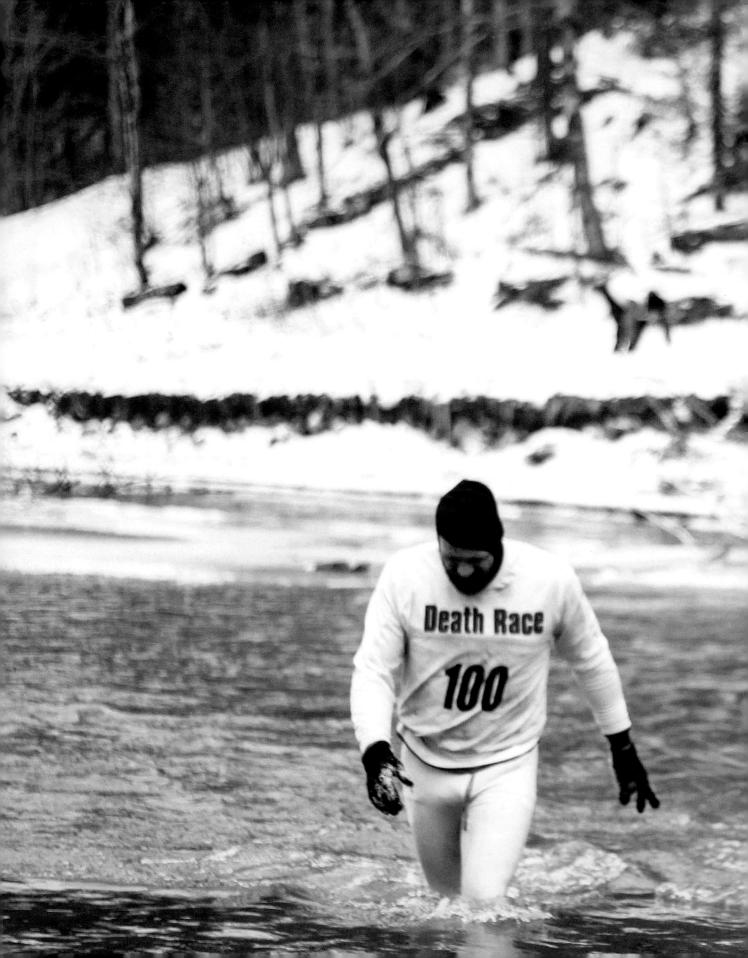

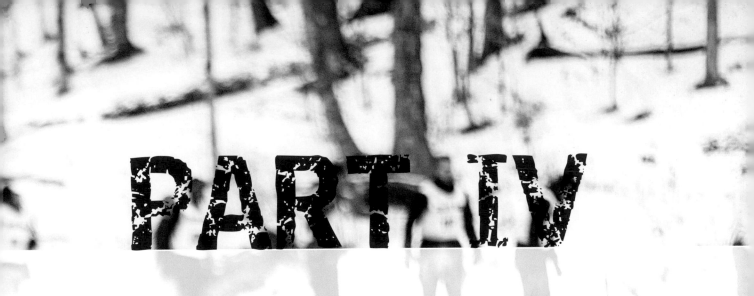

PART IV

ADVANCED OCR

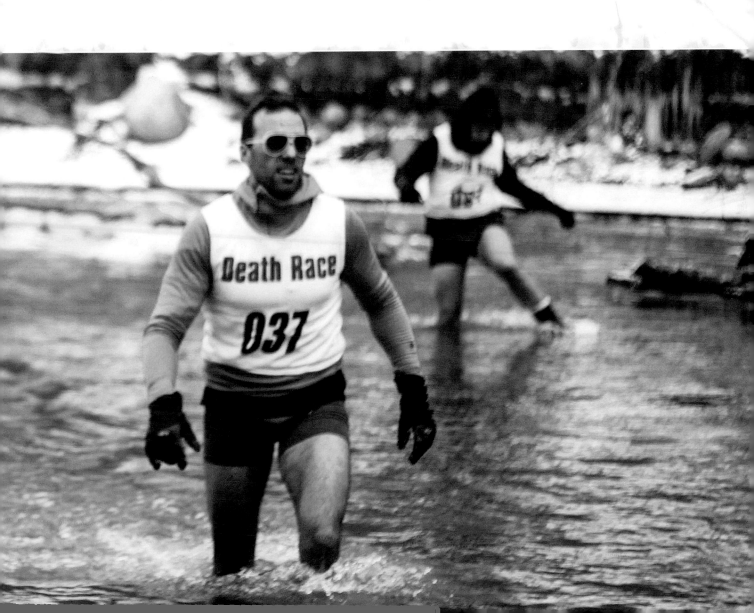

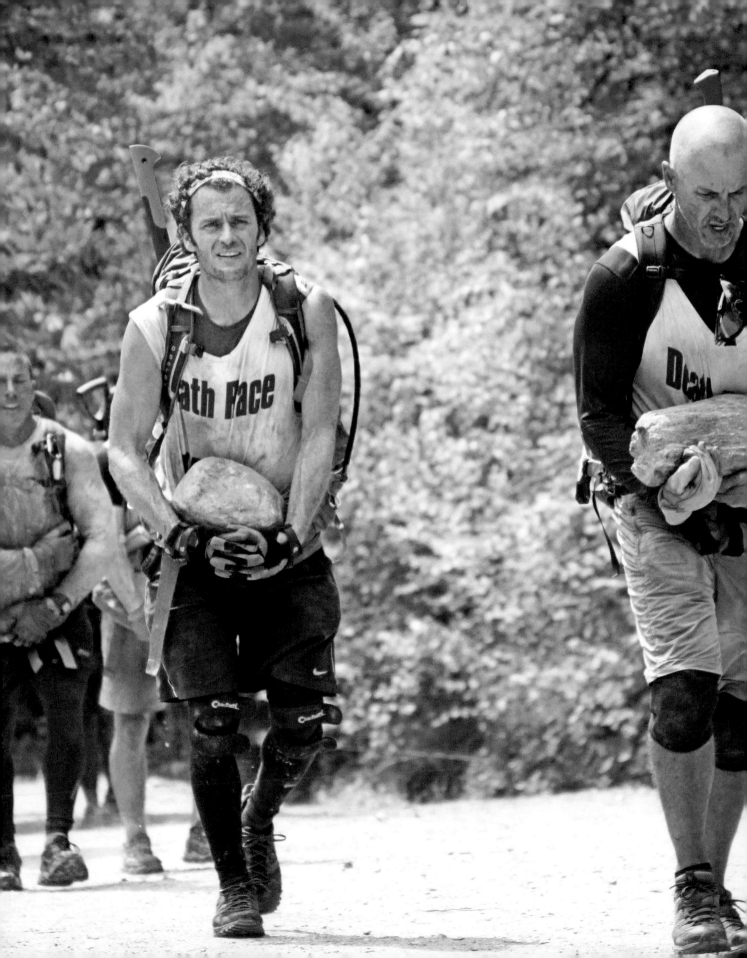

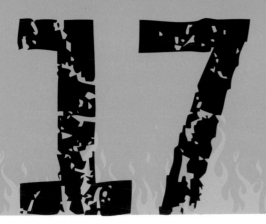

17 TRAINING FOR 24-HOUR AND ENDURANCE OCR EVENTS

☙ Featuring Amelia Boone and Olof Dallner

For this chapter on surviving 24-hour-plus events, I reached out to the best in the business. Here is a list of just some of their accomplishments:

Amelia Boone and Olof Dallner have both won the 60-plus-hour Death Race, and they have finished multiple times.

After finishing second last year in the 26-plus-mile (41.8-plus-km) obstacle race known as the Ultra Beast, Boone won it in 2013 in spectacular fashion. Dallner was the second-place male this year behind only Junyong Pak.

Additionally, Boone won World's Toughest Mudder in 2012 and almost every short distance obstacle race that she entered in 2013. Dallner, meanwhile, is one of a select few who were handpicked

for the 48-plus-hour GORUCK Selection and completed it successfully. In addition, he won the Quintuple Anvil Ultra Triathalon in just under four days.

For this chapter, I asked them both how they prepare mentally and physically to perform at such a high level for such a long period of time.

Olof, How do you increase your endurance?

Endurance is to be able to repeat an action, to remain active for a prolonged time. More important, it is the ability to endure difficulty and hardship. For many people, endurance is being able to physically perform for a certain time, such as completing a marathon.

In my mind, the mental aspect of endurance is more interesting. I grew

◄ *The Death Race will push you in ways you have never been pushed.*

up inspired by people such as Thor Heyerdahl, a Norwegian adventurer and explorer who built a primitive raft and sailed it 5,000 miles (8,000 km) across the Pacific Ocean in 101 days. He inspired me to go further and explore my limits.

Why would this have relevance to endurance obstacle racing? Often, longer obstacle races have many unknowns, or unexpected things will likely happen during the race. Some of these races are really just about finishing. It is important to be physically prepared, but you stand no chance without the right mindset. When you are at the start line, the major thing that can get in your way is your own brain. Worrying about what is out there instead of focusing on the task at hand may be your downfall. Imagine taking a step from shore onto a raft made of balsa wood to sail 5,000 miles (8,000 km) across the Pacific Ocean in 1947. There is no room for worrying about what is going to happen after 4,000 miles (6,400 km) somewhere at sea.

Olof, how do you build mental endurance?

My philosophy for building everyday mental toughness is to choose the worst circumstances for training when possible. When I used to get ready for a climbing expedition, my partner and I would pick a Sunday following a particularly party-heavy Saturday night to go climbing. Preferably it would rain, we would put on mountain boots instead of friction climbing shoes, make sure we were very sleep deprived, and then go climb a very exposed, mentally tasking route. This is a very good simulation for how you will feel high up on a mountain when you really need to perform.

> "It is important to be physically prepared, but you stand no chance without the right mindset."

This is my approach for an endurance obstacle race, too. If you are out there for a long time, the probability is exponentially higher that weather will be bad, you will be out of nutrition and water, and you will be lost and getting increasingly stressed about it. You can train for this by depriving yourself from these stressors and seeing how you react and how you perform. You will learn more about how to prepare yourself and not stress about it. Endurance is experience and knowledge.

Once you are toeing the start line, however, it's time to focus on the task at hand. It's common to worry too much about what will happen later on and not

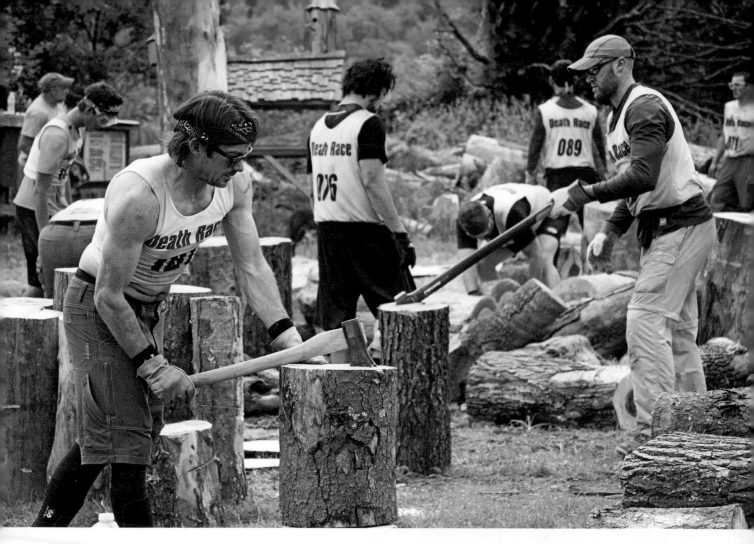

◄ *Wood chopping has become a staple at OCR endurance events.*

focus on what is in front of you right now. It is not tunnel vision but a very concentrated focus on where you are at this very minute. What are you doing at the obstacle in front of you? Where is the trail going the next 20 feet (6.1 m)?

Most elite athletes practice visualization, and there are obvious reasons for this. Seeing yourself completing something in your head is a lot better than going around talking about how you are going to do something. People who are good at visualizing perform better and are more likely to finish. So the start of the race is not where you should start second-guessing yourself. See yourself going through the entire race and finishing.

If you are in a very long endurance race with many obstacles, you're also likely to fail one or several obstacles. You may even fail all of them. This is where compartmentalization is key. What happened at a certain point in the race can be cornered off and locked into a part of

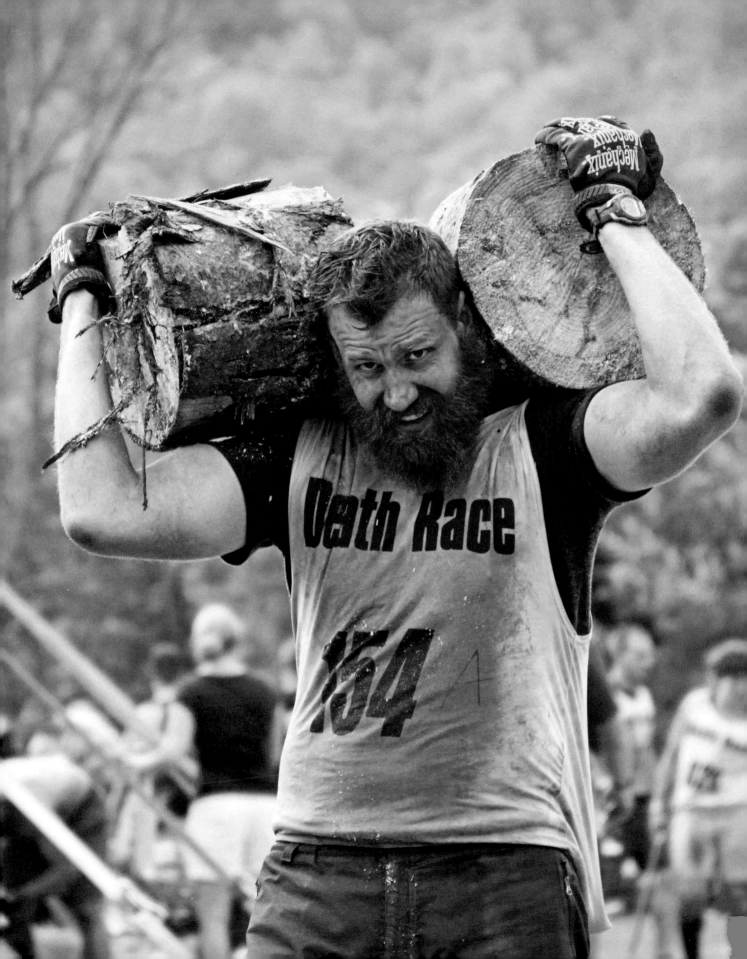

your brain. Say to yourself, "Okay, I'm done with that, did not go so well, move on." You can learn to do this efficiently, and you will fail fewer obstacles if you can do this, particularly if you get a bad start. You should not let yourself be too emotional and let that affect the rest of your race.

If you end up doing a race that is very long, maybe days, there will surely be ups and downs. Your brain wants you to stop much earlier than you really need to. That is just a protective mechanism; humans should reserve energy and power for when it is really needed. If you think you have to stop, and you really can't go further, I assure you that you would run a personal record pace if a bear suddenly decides to come after you. Experience in endurance racing will give you tools to deal with this. I think about how fortunate I am to be able to be out there and doing it. I take a look at my surroundings and smile at how beautiful things are, and usually that gives me my energy to go on.

The naysaying voices in your head get a lot worse if you did not take care of your nutrition. Countless times I have seen people quit, take a 5-minute break with some water and nutrition, and then look dumbfounded about why they actually quit. Try to keep your emotions in line and be rational. If you are having negative thoughts and thinking about quitting, take a short break and check yourself. Most of the time, you'll be back on track before you know it.

Amelia, what kind of mental attitude does it take to last 24 hours plus?

I know many endurance athletes say that you can't even let yourself consider quitting, because as soon as you do, you've already defeated yourself. I disagree. I think about quitting pretty much every 24-hour-plus race I've done. I think you're lying to yourself, or downright irresponsible, if you don't consider that, especially when your physical well-being starts to get compromised—which it will. I prefer to take the event in chunks, and I only focus on the next obstacle or next task, and no further beyond that. When you start to think about where you are in the grand scheme of things ("only three hours in?"), then you start to second-guess yourself.

You do, however, need to have a high threshold for pain and for being uncomfortable, and you need to have the ability to disengage from those feelings. But I think,

◄ *Sure this guy is huge, but a huge heart is what separates the winners at these kinds of events.*

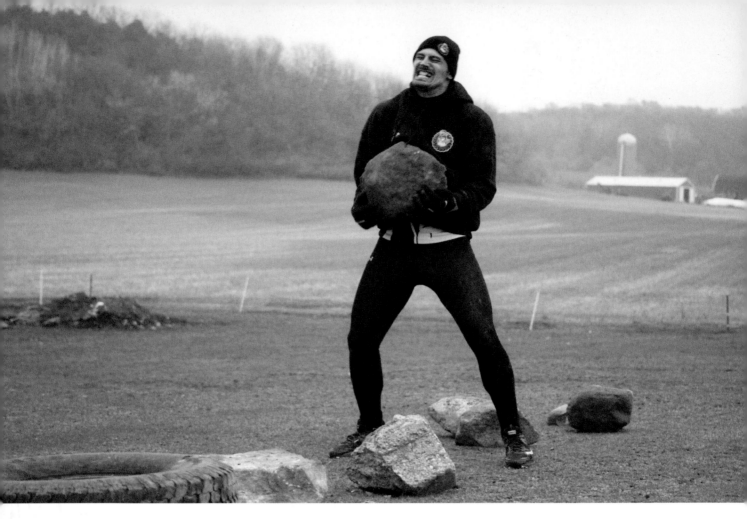

▲ *You may be asked to complete tasks alone . . .*

most important, you need to keep the fun in it for as long as possible. If you've ever seen pictures of me from races, I'm always trying to smile. And, for the most part, I have a blast. But there will come a point in the 24-hour-plus events where you will hate life, and that's natural. So find ways to have a good time while you are out there.

Olof, how do you improve your physical endurance?

There's really no secret to increasing your endurance in different disciplines. To me, it seems people need to be more honest with themselves. What's your weakness? As I mentioned before, endurance obstacle racing very often has unknown elements, and you're likely to encounter obstacles you haven't seen before. Identify your weakness and train to improve. Many athletes in this sport put emphasis on doing obstacles. But more specific exercises will result in greater improvement faster. If you're a slower runner, you will have to acknowledge this and train to be faster. Long average-tempo runs will

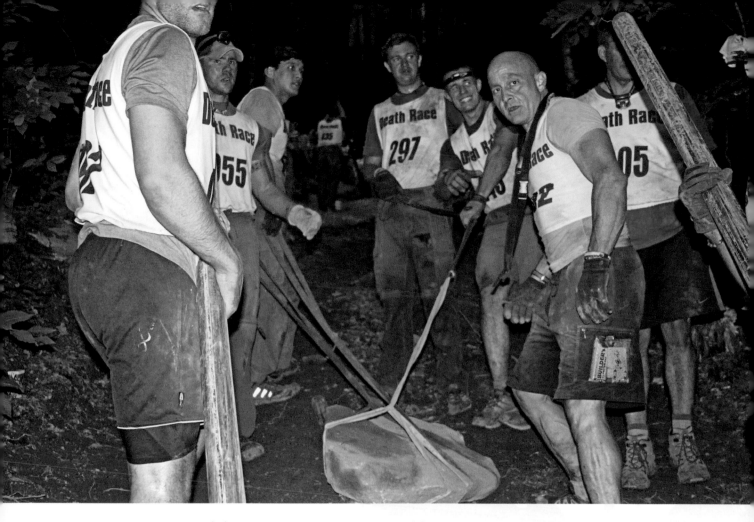

▲ . . . *or your competitors might be your teammates at certain times of the event.*

not accomplish this. You will need to do sprints and intervals, maybe even find a track to do your workouts on. If you aren't a good swimmer, you should think about improving that skill. Most obstacle races don't include a proper swim, but I'm sure it will happen, and you should be prepared for it. All of this means you need to push yourself outside your comfort zone. That does not necessarily mean you should carry a tire until you feel very uncomfortable. Does a 3- to 5-mile (4.8- to 8.1-km) swim sound like it's outside your comfort zone? It is not impossible, but it requires training, and you will have to take a step outside of said comfort zone. I personally like to train for a wide variety of things, and I try to constantly identify my weaknesses to improve on them. There is always plenty of work to be done no matter what level you are on. Don't get comfortable with just going back to do the same workout all the time.

Caring for your feet is a topic frequently discussed in these types of events. This could be an issue in a regular ultra, too,

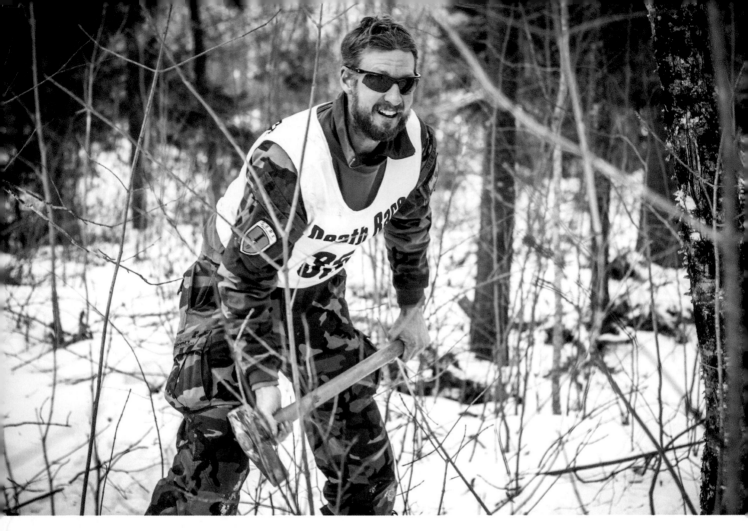

▲ *This is legendary Death Racer Todd Sedlak. Many have credited his wisdom of "nothing more than 5 minutes or 5 feet (1.5 m) ahead of you" with helping them complete the event.*

but it's a bigger factor in an obstacle endurance event. You're more likely to spend a long time being wet and muddy with little time to rest, maybe carrying something heavy, putting even more stress on your feet. Blisters and maceration will happen in no time. First and foremost, I emphasize foot strength and running form. Stronger feet in combination with a good running form will decrease the stress that your feet will experience.

Most of these races require you to stay on your feet for a long time. I do some of my run training with a focus on keeping a good running form and avoiding putting my feet too hard to the ground, using a much shorter and quicker stride. I also do some foot strengthening exercises on balance boards and one-legged balance squats. The second way to counteract the destruction of your feet is self-discipline at every little break you get. If you can dry out one foot for 20 seconds, do that.

Next break, you can dry out the other foot. If you have been up for two days straight, it's very tempting to just lean back on your backpack and sleep instead of attending to your feet. This is where self-discipline and experience come into play. You will have to think of your priorities.

Amelia, what kind of training do you specifically do for 24-hour-plus endurance events?

It's difficult to train for a 24-hour race, because you hit a point of diminishing returns. In other words, it makes no sense to do a 4- or 5-hour workout. I do CrossFit five or six days a week, and I either run, ruck, or hit the giant step mill four or five days a week. Aside from one rest day a week (which may incorporate yoga, a light jog, and mobility), I'm generally training 1.5 to 2 hours a day in a variety of disciplines.

Amelia, how does your "endurance event" training (World's Toughest Mudder, Death Race) differ from your "regular" or OCR training?

Aside from the fact that I actually will taper for a few days before a long race, my training doesn't vary at all. I try to keep my body in peak physical condition year-round, which is all you can really do to train for a race that lasts a day or more. At some point, the race shifts from the physical to the mental.

Amelia, what kind of physical shape should racers be in before they attempt 24-hour-plus events? Can anyone do them?

Can anyone do them? Sure. *Should* anyone do them? Probably not. Honestly, *no one* should do 24-hour-plus events. But I'm a firm believer that people give up mentally before they give up physically in these 24-hour-plus events. The first WTM, none of us had any idea what to expect. I had only done two Tough Mudders previously. How I survived and finished—and came in second—but others quit after a lap or two likely isn't explained by lack of physical preparation. Anyone can really do them, as long as you go in with realistic expectations of what to expect your first time. You may "blow up" and DNF [did not finish], or you may surprise yourself and win. Some people are suited for the long haul, but others aren't. There's no way of knowing which you are until you attempt it.

Olof, what are your thoughts on nutrition for longer endurance races?

The longer the race, the less dependent I try to be on fast nutrition such as energy

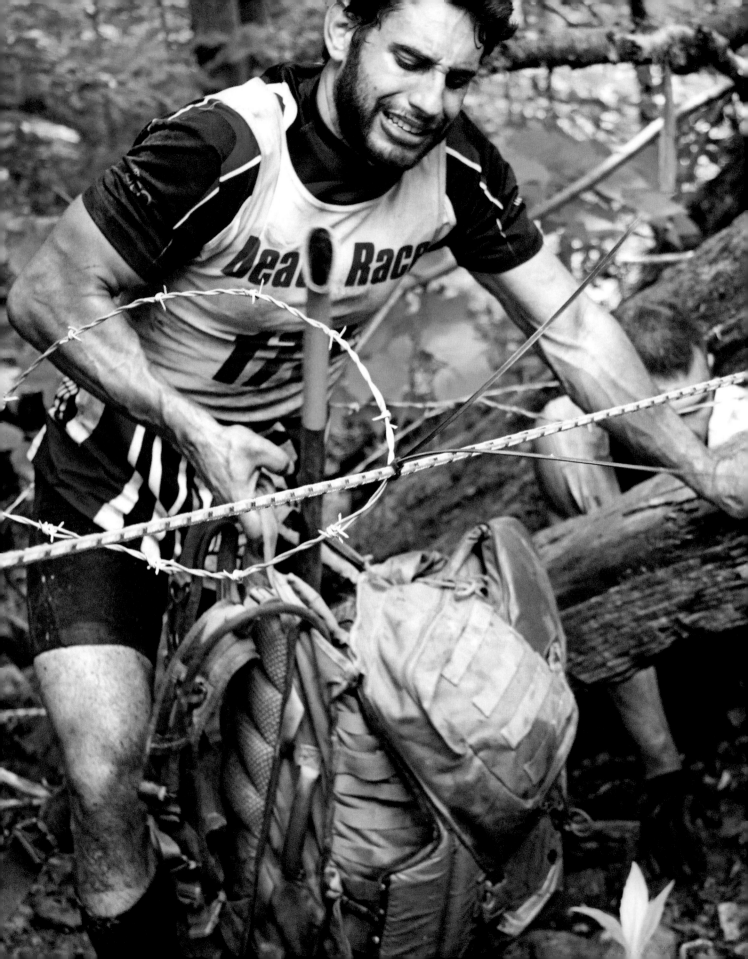

gels. Stretching over days, I prefer to eat regular meals with snacks in between. It is really a very personal preference about what works for you, and you will need to figure that out. The golden rule is: Don't try something new on race day. I find that if it's possible to have access to liquid nutrition such as a fruit/vegetable smoothie, I'm able to consume more calories quicker without upsetting my stomach.

Try to keep some of your nutrition close at hand. If you pack all of your nutrition in your backpack, you're more likely to skip taking in some nutrition often. That could result in one of the previously mentioned mental down turns when you feel like quitting. When that happens, first eat and drink something that you have in your pocket. During a very long race, you're more prone to losing electrolytes, so bringing salt/electrolyte pills works for most people.

Depriving yourself of nutrition and water during training does not really adapt your body to it, but it could help you with the mental aspect of pushing through. If you are looking to train to improve your physical fitness and endurance, you should not do this. Decide what your plan is for the event and then just let it go. People tend to overthink what type of energy bar to bring or what electrolytes. Most of the time, it will have very little impact on the outcome—unless you forgot to bring it entirely!

Amelia, what are your thoughts on nutrition? Has it changed for you recently from other types of training?
I'm eating Milk Duds right now as I write this. Seriously. Generally, I eat a Paleo/Primal diet, but I find my body operates better with more carbs than those diets typically recommend, and I'm a sucker for ice cream and ketchup —not together. I used to pray before the high-carb, low-fat "altar," so adding fats and focusing on proteins and veggies has been a shift.

A few days before races, I increase my carb intake. But during long races, everything goes out the window. You never know what your stomach will be able to handle during long races, or what is going to sound appealing, so I bring a variety. When I won WTM 2012, I was mainly fueled by Pedialyte, Ensure, and Pop-Tarts. I don't recommend it, but it got me through.

◄ *How you pack can make or break your endurance event success.*

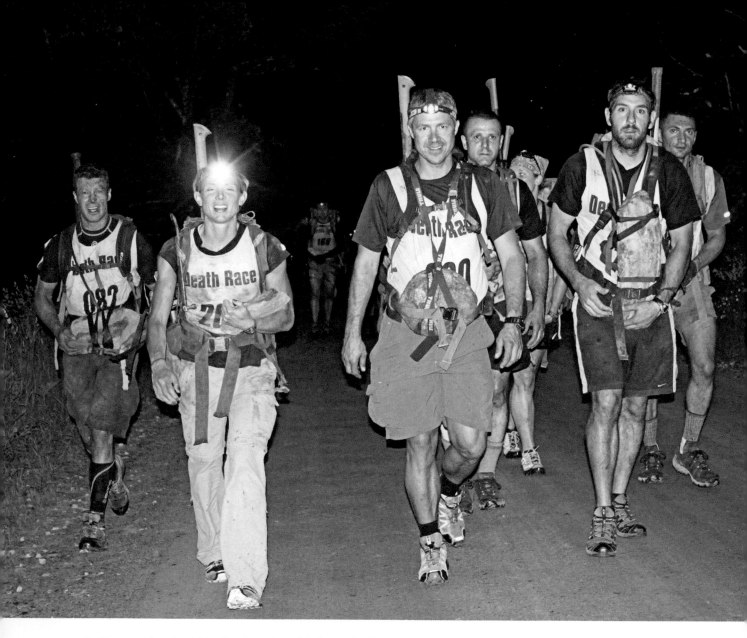

▲ *Your packing should be simple and straightforward. That way when it's dark and your brain isn't working at its peak performance, you'll still be able to find what you need to refuel and revive.*

Amelia, how important is gear selection in planning for 24-hour-plus events?

Admittedly, endurance events, especially cold-weather ones, tend to be very gear-intensive, but there's a fine line between having things organized/having everything you need and obsessing over or becoming overly dependent on your gear.

I'm an over-packer in life, so I tend to be for races as well, but I find that I generally don't use everything I bring. For instance, I didn't change clothes or shoes once during WTM last year. On the other hand, I didn't bring a handsaw to the 2012 Summer Death Race, and I was kicking myself for all three days.

In general, you want to look for light, packable gear that can multitask. For instance, for winter events, think wool, and make sure you have your extremities covered. For summer events, always bring extra electrolyte tabs and hydration. Some endurance races will allow you to bring a bin or drop box for extra supplies.

> "I didn't bring a handsaw to the 2012 Summer Death Race, and I was kicking myself for all three days."

If you do bring one, organization is key. Some people prefer to pack their nutrition in individual plastic zip-top bags so they can just grab one and go. I always label and sort the day before so I know where everything is. Inevitably, mid-race, most likely in the middle of the night, things will get shuffled around, so it's important to try to control that from the beginning.

When Amelia Boone is not running obstacle or endurances races, she is an attorney in Chicago, Illinois. She typically updates her blog at http://raceipsa.blogspot.com after she wins something. She also famously enjoys ketchup.

DOWN AND DIRTY TAKEAWAYS

- **Improve on skills that need practice.** Work on the things that you're naturally not good at. It's the only way to get better.
- **Find nutrition and gear plans and stick with them.** While training, try various nutrition and gear options. Figure out what works for you, and do not change it on race day. Don't worry once you're settled with your plan, just go with it. It is going to suck anyway.
- **Recreate bad days.** Train in poor conditions when possible to simulate race day hardships.
- **Organize ahead of time.** Things will get shuffled on the day, so the easier to find things in the middle of the night, the better. Make it idiot-proof so when your brain is not at 100 percent, you can find the things that will help you get right again.
- **Do not quit.** Learn to check yourself and keep your emotions in line. Remember that the voice in your head will be deceptive.

Olof Dallner is a Swedish national currently living in New York City, pursuing scientific research at Rockefeller University. He has a PhD in physiology, and he has made cheap sunglasses cool in the ultra-endurance community.

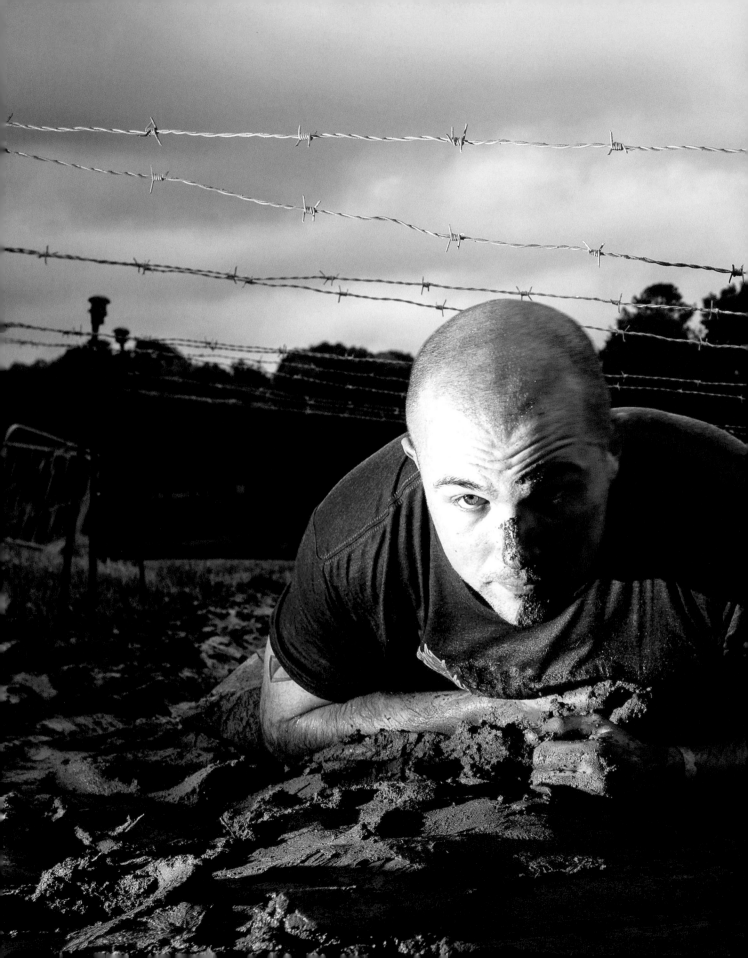

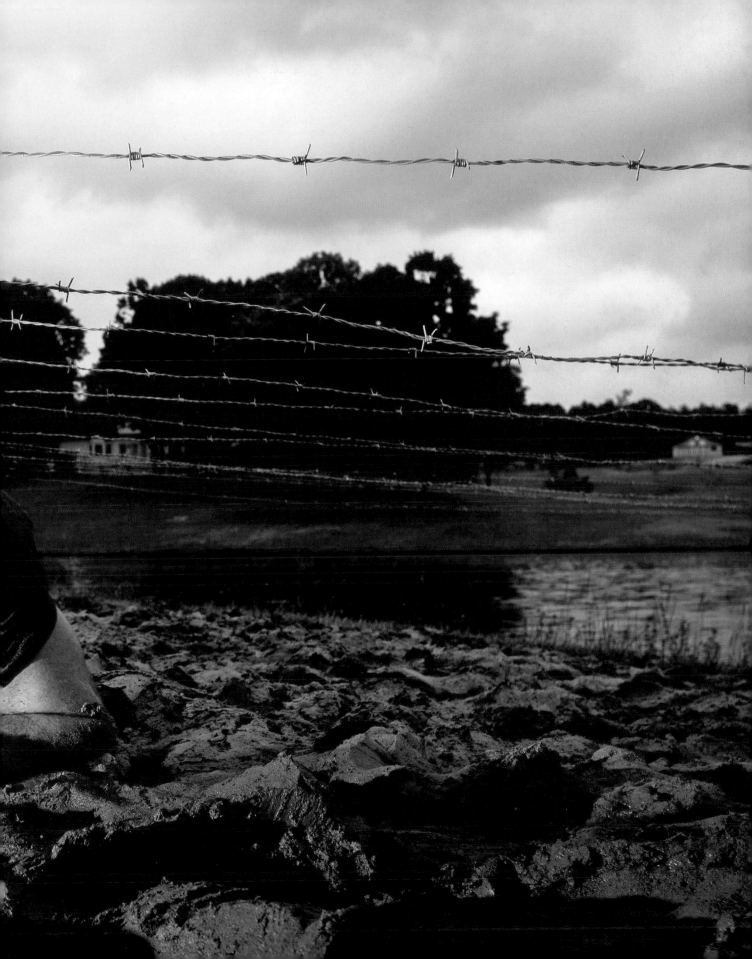

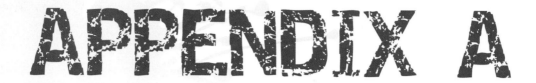

APPENDIX A

OCR COMMUNITIES

AZN ARMOUR IN FLORIDA AND OTHER STATES:
Contact Jay Tea at jaymestran@yahoo.com. Visit www.facebook.com/groups/AznArmour.

CANADIAN MUDD QUEENS: Contact Sara Logan at maneensl@hotmail.com.
Visit www.facebook.com/groups/MuddQueens and www.MuddQueens.blogspot.com.

CHICAGO SPARTANS IN ILLINOIS:
Contact Paul Sutfin at TeamChicagoSpartan@gmail.com.
Visit www.facebook.com/groups/MuddQueens and www.MuddQueens.blogspot.com.

COLORADO OBSTACLE RACERS: Contact Leslie St. Louis at
ColoradoObstacleRacers.com@gmail.com. Visit www.facebook.com/
ColoradoObstacleRacersPage, www.coloradoobstacleracers.com,
Twitter: @ColoradoOCR, and www.facebook.com/groups/CORAllProEPCBeasts.

CORN FED SPARTANS IN INDIANA AND THE MIDWEST: Contact Jonathan Nolan
at jnolan@cornfedspartans.com. Visit www.facebook.com/CornFedSpartan,
www.cornfedspartans.com, and Twitter: @CornFedSpartans.

CRAZY MUDDER MUCKERS IN KENTUCKY, OHIO, WEST VIRGINIA, AND INDIANA:
Contact Kevin Jones at kjones@crazymuddermuckers.com.
Visit www.facebook.com/groups/crazymuddermuckers and www.crazymudder
muckers.com.

GEORGIA OBSTACLE RACERS & MUD RUNNERS (GORMR): Contact Delaine Anderson at
s.delaine.anderson@gmail.com. Visit www.facebook.com/groups/GORMR.

HOUSTON TOUGH MUDDERS IN TEXAS:
Contact Willie Vera at willie_vera@yahoo.com. Visit www.facebook.com/groups/
HoustonToughmudders, Twitter: @slawburb, and Instagram: slawburb.

LONE STAR SPARTANS IN TEXAS: Contact Paul Almanza at lonestarspartansocr@gmail.
com. Visit www.facebook.com/lonestarspartans, www.lonestarspartans.com,
Twitter: @LSSOCR, and Instagram: Lone Star Spartans.

MIDWEST VIKINGS: Contact Tata Fenwick at tata@midwestvikings.com.
Visit www.facebook.com/groups/midwestvikings, www.midwestvikings.com,
Twitter: @MidwestVikings, and www.facebook.com/midwestvikings.

NEW ENGLAND SPAHTENS: Contact Paul Jones at paul@nespahtens.com. Visit
www.facebook.com/nespahtens, http://join.nespahtens.com, Twitter: @nespahtens,
and Pinterest: nespahtens.

PA O.C.R. KEYSTONESPARTANS IN PENNSYLVANIA: Contact Michael Matter at
mmatter@pa.gov. Visit www.facebook.com/groups/262051050523231/.

TEAM BRAVEHEART IN NEW YORK, NEW JERSEY, AND CONNECTICUT:
Contact Jen Rosant at teambraveheartllc@gmail.com. Visit www.facebook.com/
BeBraveTeamBraveheart and www.braveheartathletics.com.

TEAM MUDRUNFUN IN FLORIDA AND OTHER STATES: Contact Damion Trombley at
damion@mudrunfun.com or matthew@mudrunfun.com.
Visit www.facebook.com/mudrunfun, www.mudrunfun.com,
Twitter: @mudrunfun, and www.mudrunfun.com/magazine.

TEAM SISU ON THE WEST COAST:
Contact Matt Trinca at matt@sisuteam.com.
Visit www.facebook.com/groups/teamsisu, www.sisuteam.com,
and Twitter: @Team_SISU1.

WEEPLE ARMY ON THE WEST COAST: Contact Dave Huckle at weeplearmy@gmail.com.
Visit www.facebook.com/groups/WeepleArmy, www.WeepleArmy.com, and
Twitter: @WeepleArmy.

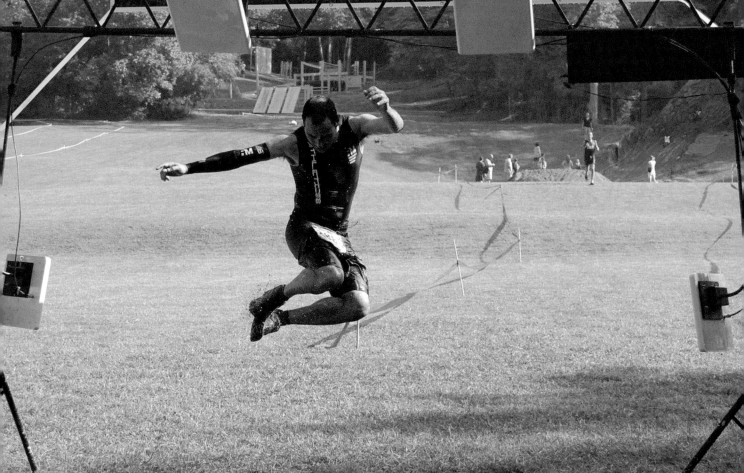

APPENDIX B

OCR RESOURCES

WEBSITES
- www.obstacleracingmedia.com
- www.mudrunfun.com
- www.mudrunguide.com
- www.travlete.com
- www.mudandadventure.com
- www.obstacleracemagazine.com (UK)
- www.obstacleracers.com.au (Australia)

BLOGGERS TO FOLLOW
- www.dirtinyourskirt.com: Margaret Schlachter
- www.relentlessforwardcommotion.com: Heather Gannoe
- www.dankrueger.net: Dan Krueger
- www.funkyfitnesspdx.com: Katrina "Ninjarina" Blackwell
- www.onmywaytosparta.com: Dr. Jeff Cain
- www.legendofthedeathrace.com: Anthony Matesi
- www.muddymommy.com: Holly Joy Berkey
- www.barbwireforbreakfast.com: Andi Hardy, Corrine Kohlen, and Ang Reynolds
- www.raceipsa.blogspot.com: Amelia Boone
- www.mudmanreport.com: Kevin LaPlatney
- www.solovieva.com: Ekaterina "Solo" Solovieva

PODCASTS
- Obstacle Racing Media Podcast hosted by Matt B. Davis: http://obstacleracingmedia.com/podcast
- Getting Dirty Podcast with Daniel and Laurie: www.gettingdirtypodcast.com

YOUTUBE TO FOLLOW
- Inside Obstacle News
- JWatson TV

◄ *My last pieces of advice: Always finish in style, and always know where the camera is.*

INDEX

Note: <u>Underscored</u> page references indicate boxed text. **Boldface** page references indicate photographs.

PHOTOGRAPHER CREDITS

Adam Berkey, 10; 21; 24; 33; 39; 43; 49; 52; 57; 61; 69; 122; 124; 125; 129; 134; 158; 159; 171; 61

Donald Chambers, 160; 163; 165; 167; 170; 172

Paul Jones/New England Spahtens, 60; 140; 147; 152

Madmotion, 198; 201; 202; 205; 208; 210

Anthony J. Matesi, 86; 102; 104; 118; 120; 196–197; 204; 206

Mud Guts and Glory/Hosted by King's Domain, 63; 65; 75; 76; 77; 84; 98; 106; 130; 136; 216

Bob Mulholland, 18; 58

Tim Nettleton/TrueSpeedPhoto.com, 189 (top)

Nuvision Action Image, 224

Race Pace Photos, 7; 8–9; 12; 15; 16–17; 23; 26; 28; 30; 34; 36; 41; 44; 51; 53; 54; 66; 78; 80; 83; 88–89; 90; 92; 95; 97; 116; 126–127; 132; 139; 144; 148; 150–151; 156; 184; 212–213

Dana Rasmussen, 109; 110; 111; 113; 114

Vince Rhee/New England Spahtens, 46; 70; 72; 143

Richard Ricciardi, 189 (bottom)

David Young/Coast Shots Photography, LLC, 174; 177; 178; 181

ACKNOWLEDGMENTS

I will start with all of the amazing athletes, race directors, and photographers who contributed to this book. Next, I want to thank my editor, Jess Haberman, whom I drove slightly more than crazy during this whole process.

In addition, I would like to thank Doug Grady and Dominic Carubba, who inspired me to tackle that first Tough Mudder. Chris LePage, my neighbor who became my first running partner, Wes Kaye, who was my first running mentor. Andi Hardy who made me my first sandbag and helped me to start our local, amazing OCR group— Georgia Obstacle Racers and Mud Runners (GORMR). Carissa Worm, Clint Turner and the Decatur Running Club. Aaron Moss, Matt Ross, TJ Pitts and the End of Days Run Club.

Thanks to Joe Desena, Andy Weinberg, Carrie Adams, Mike Morris, Tommy Mac, and everyone from Spartan who has always been kind, open, and accessible. Bob Babbitt and everyone at Competitor. Lindsay Babb, Greg Lang and the rest of the wackos over at Hard Charge, Alex Patterson, Cristina Devito, and everyone at Tough Mudder. Ken Park, John King, Brad Cousino and everyone who works at Mud, Guts and Glory, Sam Abbitt and everyone at Savage, Adam McDonald from the original Obstacle Racing Magazine, Sean O'Connor and everyone at Superhero Scramble, Josue Stephens and his entire family from FuegoYAuga Events. Ike Murov and everyone at Red Frog Events. The Heads of the 5 Families. Paul Jones from New England Spahtens, Damion and Tracy from Trombley from MudRunFun, Dave Huckle from the Weeple Army, Jonathan Nolan from Cornfed, and Kevin Jones from Crazy Mudder Muckers.

I'd like to thank Ray Upshaw for giving me my first amazing interview and a podcast episode that people still talk about.

Thanks to Scott Keneally for being the only guy I could turn to about a million times and for the movie you are going to make.

Some folks did additional research and helped finalize important details without which, this book would not have been finished. They are James Megliola, Amy Lillis, and Desiree Rincon.

I called every published author I knew and bugged them to death with questions. They are Suzy Soro, Kyria Abrahams, Tonio Andrade, Eric Orton, Brett Stewart, and Margaret Schlachter.

The Obstacle Racing Media Team. First and foremost Christian "Cranky" Griffith aka C$: The best partner anyone could have. Also Valerie Hinsley, Alex "ThunderDart" Martin, Hope Epton, and Kaitlin Stein.

My brothers across the water: James Musgrave in Australia and Carl Wibberly and Peter Rees in the U.K.

I'd like to thank you, because you most likely helped me over a wall, gave me a ride to a race, got me unstuck from some barbed wire, or allowed me to do the same for you.

Last but not least, I would like to thank my family. My wife, Stacie: Honey, you are the most supportive human being a husband could ask for. Also, my kids Emma, Jaxson, and River: You remind me every day of what is really important.

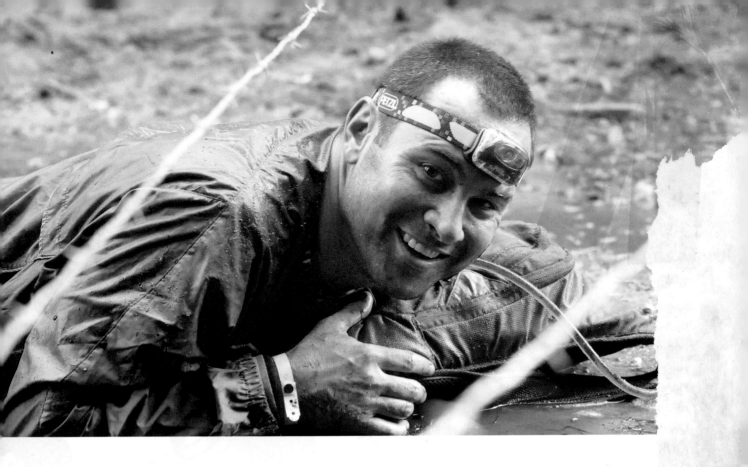

ABOUT THE AUTHOR

Matt B. Davis is a journalist and podcaster who specializes in obstacle course racing and mud runs. He has completed more than fifty events of every distance and difficulty level. Through the Obstacle Racing Media website (ObstacleRacingMedia.com) and podcast, Matt has interviewed more than 100 athletes, race directors, and other OCR insiders. He lives in Atlanta, Georgia, with his wife and three child